PAIN & PERFORMANCE

PAIN
&
PERFORMANCE

The Revolutionary New Way to Use Training
as Treatment for Pain and Injury

Ryan Whited

& Matt Fitzgerald

PUBLISHING

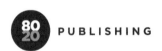 PUBLISHING

80/20 Publishing, LLC
1916 N 1150 E Lehi, UT 84043
www.8020books.com

Library of Congress Control Number: 2023945862

ISBN 979-8-9853980-4-5

Cover design by Hopewell Design
Cover photo: James Q Martin

To my mom and dad, who taught me the comeback as a way of life—a lesson that I will pass on to my son, Lane.

—Ryan

Contents

Acknowledgments

I am hopeful that *Pain & Performance* will be a catalyst to change how we care for individuals who are experiencing pain and injuries. If it weren't for the shared thoughts, research, and graciousness of some educators, scholars, and online groups, the paradigm of care would never shift. I am incredibly thankful for the shared wisdom of Bronnie Lennox Thompson, Lars Avemarie, Greg Lehman, Adam Meakins, and so many others making the change. To Matt Fitzgerald, I am extremely grateful for your intellectual curiosity and willingness to dive into this topic with me.

Furthermore, while it wasn't my intention to become obsessed with care, the deeper I went, the deeper I went. I can say that I am glad to have learned all that I have in my autodidactic journey, but it wasn't without a good deal of sacrifice. This sacrifice was shared by my family, and I'm sad to say that at one point of the journey, my phone recognized my office location as "home" because of the amount of time I spent there studying and working.

Without my wife Betsy's understanding, patience, and continual sound counseling, none of this could have ever happened. For this I'll be forever grateful.

Ryan Whited

Foreword

As a physiotherapist, chiropractor, and strength and conditioning specialist treating musculoskeletal disorders within a biopsychosocial model, I am incredibly envious of this book that Ryan Whited has written and wish that it was my own. He has done a tremendous job of weaving together the science of pain, injury, and performance and personal anecdotes to make this topic relevant to almost everyone. *Pain and Performance* is for clinicians, coaches, athletes, and pretty much anyone with a body.

In the professions Ryan and I work in, we have been hoping for a shift in how pain, injury, and performance are viewed—a move away from a very reductionistic biomedical approach. A new science-based understanding of pain and injury is needed, and this book provides a great framework for that mindset. Ryan lays a foundation for people in pain to truly understand what influences pain and injury and what we can all do to recover. A mix of engaging personal and professional stories alongside research on pain and injury gives the reader a clear view of the author's evolution as a patient, coach, and clinician.

Those in pain will see themselves in many of the clinical stories, and clinicians will see a path to helping those same people in pain. *Patient-centered care* is a buzzword in our fields, and it starts with an understanding of why we hurt. As a clinician, I would want all my patients to read *Pain and Performance*, as their doing so would enable me to become a better partner in understanding and exploring the different options available for their recovery.

Pragmatically, this is best manifested in Ryan's "Training as Treatment" mantra. Ryan has blurred the lines and even erased the unnecessary distinction between injury treatment and performance training. His experience has led him to recognize that when it comes to pain, everything matters, and the person in pain is not only a partner in their own care but a valuable resource.

I recommend *Pain and Performance* to anyone working with people in pain, anyone who is in pain, and anyone who wants to better understand human function and resiliency.

Dr. Greg Lehman, BKin, MS, DC, MScPT

Introduction

Have you ever learned something that instantly validated a whole chunk of your experience, making sense of life events that had defied all previous efforts to explain and assuring you that you weren't crazy after all? That's what meeting Ryan Whited was like for me.

It happened at Paragon Athletics, a training facility that Ryan and his wife, Betsy, operate in Flagstaff, Arizona. I showed up there on a Friday evening in October 2019 as a participant in a running camp hosted by champion ultrarunner Rob Krar, a client of Ryan's who'd asked him to deliver a presentation titled "Pain and Performance" for an audience that, in addition to Rob's campers, included a diverse mix of local athletes and healthcare professionals. I didn't know anything about Ryan before I walked in the door, but his words and slides blew my mind and subsequently transformed my athletic experience.

I like to say that no runner my age has ever suffered more injuries than I have—an unprovable claim, but probably not far from the truth. It's not that I'm accident-prone or have a low pain tolerance or take a lot of stupid risks in my training. I just have a propensity for breakdowns, particularly in my joints, that may be genetically rooted—I've seen research suggesting that athletes in whose tendons a certain type of collagen is predominant get hurt a lot. Whatever the underlying cause, I've suffered more than my fair share of minor injuries in my long career as an endurance athlete as well as three major ones—right knee, left Achilles tendon, right hip—that have kept me out of racing for more than a year apiece. Different in most respects, these three protracted injuries had one thing in common, which is that none of the obvious healing and treatment measures applied to them helped. Everything from rest to manual therapy to surgery didn't work. What ultimately *did* work, in each case, was the very thing that seemed to have caused the injury: exercise.

If it had only happened once, I probably would have dismissed the phenomenon as a fluke. If it had happened twice, I might have called it a coincidence. But three times is a pattern, and in fact, I've seen the same pattern play out with a number of my lesser injuries as well. Eventually, I decided not to even bother calling my health insurer when some part of my anatomy started to hurt, choosing instead to heal myself by training around and through the issue as my symptoms allowed, and it is a decision I do not regret. By the time I had my mind blown by Ryan Whited at the age of 48, I was losing much less training time to injuries than I had in my 20s.

Effective Treatment Options for Musculoskeletal Pain in Primary Care: A Systematic Overview of Current Evidence

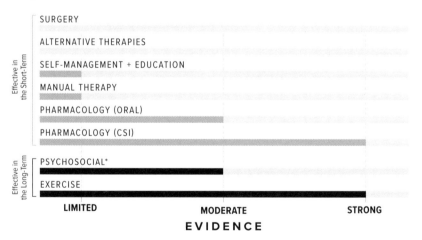

*E.g., cognitive behavioral therapy, pain coping skills training

Note: Study focused on five most common musculoskeletal pain presentations: back, neck, shoulder, knee, and multisite pain.

Source: *PLOS One* 2017 Jun 22;12(6).

The specific thing about Ryan's presentation that blew my mind is encapsulated in a graphic he shared. Adapted from a study published in the online journal *PLOS One*, it summarizes the latest scientific research on what does and what doesn't work to treat nontraumatic musculoskeletal injuries, and as you see, it jibes quite well with my personal experience.

When I saw this slide and listened to Ryan explain it, I realized I wasn't crazy after all, some bug-eyed endorphin junkie who'd convinced himself of the self-serving notion that exercise is the best way to overcome exercise-related pain. Nor was I a freak, the only athlete on earth for whom exercise really *was* the best way to overcome exercise-related pain. On the contrary, according to Ryan—and to the science on which his beliefs are based—this surprising truth is true for everyone. With obvious passion, Ryan told us he's on a mission to "demedicalize" the management of athletic pain and to treat injured athletes as *athletes*, not patients, replacing therapists with coaches and therapy with training.

Training as Treatment is Ryan's name for the systematic method he's developed to treat exercise-related pain and injury through exercise. My fellow campers and I got a taste of it the day after his talk, when we returned to Paragon to sweat our way through a series of unfamiliar yet fun exercises, many of which Ryan himself invented to help athletes train through and around pain.

I returned home to California inspired to put what I'd learned into practice and thereby take my own informal method of self-managing athletic pain to the next level. For starters, I stopped referring to myself as "injury-prone." During his talk, Ryan had explained the importance of what he called *pain self-efficacy*, or belief in one's ability to manage pain and steer the recovery process. By the same logic, I gave up familiar crutches such as nonsteroidal anti-inflammatory drugs (NSAIDs) and muscle taping, putting all my chips on Training as Treatment techniques, including graded exposure and symptom management, to get on track and stay on track with my training.

It so happened that I was dealing with a flare-up of my old hip injury at the time of my encounter with Ryan. By relying on his approach, I was able to return to full training in time for the start of the 2020 racing season, which turned out to be one of the most successful and injury-free years I've had. I ran my fastest half-marathon in 11 years, finished 14th overall and 1st in my age group at the Atlanta Marathon, ran my fastest mile since high school, and set a new personal best for 10K at age 49. Honestly, if someone had told me at the beginning of the season that I would accomplish all of this by year's end, I would have said it wasn't possible. The fact that I did wasn't a matter of defying Father Time or achieving miracles, however. I had simply discovered what is possible for any athlete who's able to stay healthy for an extended period of time.

The year was not without its hiccups. In late July, while attempting to set a marathon personal record (PR) in a small event in San Jose, California, I strained some tendons in my left foot. The silver lining to this setback was that it afforded me the opportunity to experience what it's like to work one-on-one with Ryan (remotely, via FaceTime). Right away, I was struck by how different Ryan's approach was from that of the many physical therapists, chiropractors, and other clinicians I'd seen for past injuries. Instead of prescribing a one-size-fits-all rehabilitation program to address the ankle-mobility limitation that had contributed to the injury, Ryan asked me how motivated I was for the process, explaining that he didn't want to stress me out or set me up for failure by giving me too much. I assured him that with the duathlon national championship looming, I was highly motivated to do whatever it took to return to full training as quickly as possible, and with Ryan's help, I was able to do so within three weeks. What's more, those three weeks during which I was not able to train normally were far less anxiety filled than they would have been without the tools I learned from Ryan. I felt more in control of my situation and less burdened by uncertainty.

By this time, Ryan and I were already well along in the process of writing this book, having first discussed the idea of working together a few weeks after I came home from Rob Krar's camp. We were well matched: Ryan had the message, I had writing experience, and we now shared his conviction that the product of our collaboration would meet an urgent need in the athlete community. As both an athlete and a coach, I know that pain and injury are universal experiences not just in my main sport of running but also in Ryan's sport of climbing and every other sport you can name. I also know that very few athletes are aware of the Training as Treatment method of musculoskeletal care or the new science of pain it's based on—heck, it took me several decades and a little dumb luck to find them myself! And now, with this book, *you've* found them, and I'm confident that what you learn in the pages ahead will transform your athletic experience for the better, just as my mind-blowing experience in Ryan's facility did for me.

Less pain, fewer injuries, less downtime from training, fewer visits to clinicians, less anxiety about pain and injury, less time and money wasted on treatments that don't work, better performance, and a more fulfilling athletic journey. . . . How does all that sound? I thought so. Let's make it happen!

Matt Fitzgerald, coauthor

THE GIFT OF PAIN

A few years ago, a leading over-the-counter pain medicine ran an advertising campaign targeting athletes and exercisers. In a series of 30-second television spots, everyday men and women were shown grimacing through group fitness classes as the voice-over intoned the brand's market-tested tagline: "When pain says you can't, Advil says you can."

Millions of athletes and fitness enthusiasts saw these ads and thought nothing of them. But for me, a trainer dedicated to helping athletes self-manage pain, the new slogan encapsulated what's wrong with how pain is taught and treated today. And what's wrong with it is, well, everything.

PAIN IS NORMAL

For starters, contrary to what you've always been told, pain is normal. It has existed for as long as organisms with nervous systems have existed and is an inescapable part of being alive. Only in modern times, when everything that can possibly be medicalized has been medicalized, has pain come to be regarded as pathological—something you need a pill for.

Yes, pain is unpleasant, but *unpleasant* is not synonymous with *bad*. In *feeling* bad, pain serves the crucial purpose of signaling threats (like when a painfully loud noise warns you of potential harm to your eardrums) and motivates self-protective actions (like covering your ears to block out that loud noise). It's natural to avoid pain, but you sure as heck wouldn't want to take a pill that made you incapable of feeling it. People who suffer from congenital insensitivity to pain *can't feel it*, and they often die prematurely because they're unable to take self-protective measures when threats to their well-being arise.

For athletes, pain serves the additional purpose of marking physical limits. Similar to fatigue, pain lets an athlete know when they are approaching the edge of their body's current capacity. Developing as an athlete requires a delicate balance between respecting and challenging limits, and pain is an essential tool in maintaining this balance. I tell athletes to think of pain as their employee, not their employer. If you employ pain appropriately, you will find more success and greater fulfillment as an athlete than you would if you let it boss you around. In my gym, pain doesn't say, "You can't"—it says, "Proceed with caution," or, "Let's try something slightly different."

Pain Is Not Synonymous with Injury

Most athletes associate pain with tissue damage. That's because they've been taught to do so by doctors, physical therapists, and other clinicians educated in the so-called structural model of pain, where pain is thought to be directly caused by underlying tissue damage, which is in turn caused by incorrect movement patterns, which are in turn caused by imbalances in the musculoskeletal system. In reality, the link between pain and injury is a lot looser than we've been led to believe. People often experience pain in a part of the body that has no significant underlying tissue damage, and just as often, we experience little or no pain in parts that do have significant damage. That's why the International Association for the Study of Pain now defines pain as an "unpleasant sensory and emotional experience associated with, or resembling that associated with, actual or potential tissue damage." Yet the medical establishment continues to conflate pain and injury, a stubborn error that results in overdiagnosis, overtreatment, and iatrogenic pain, or pain caused by unnecessary medical intervention.

To be clear, tissue damage frequently does contribute to pain experiences, but it is never the singular cause of pain. In 1977, physician and psychiatrist George Engel introduced a new *biopsychosocial* model of pain in which pain was understood to be fluid, personal, and multidimensional and influenced by biology, psychology, and the social context. Initially dismissed by the medical establishment, this model has gained traction in recent years, although the structural model remains dominant.

One example of a psychological factor that affects pain experience is *expectancy*. Simply put, people tend to feel pain when they expect pain. This has been shown in a variety of studies, including one by Norwegian researchers involving subjects who believed (as many people do) that the radio waves emitted by cell phones gave them headaches. Sure enough, when these individuals were exposed to radio waves in a laboratory setting, a majority reported experiencing headaches. However, they reported the same symptoms when they were merely *told* they were being exposed to radio waves and in fact were not!

Unfortunately for athletes and exercisers, today's standard process for treating workout-related pain remains based on outdated ideas about pain that originated with René Descartes in the 17th century rather than on the biopsychosocial model. Among the many problems with the current treatment process is that it creates poor expectancies. Consider the typical sequence of events that unfolds when an athlete experiences pain that's significant and persistent enough to interfere with training.

First, the athlete is likely to assume that the pain is being caused by an injury because, again, athletes have been conditioned to do just that. As I've suggested, though, pain often occurs in the absence of an underlying injury, and to assume that something must be wrong whenever pain reaches a certain level of intensity and persistence can lead to negative consequences. Evidence of these consequences comes from research involving Aboriginal cultures where the medicalization of pain is less prevalent. A study conducted by Israeli researchers and published in the journal *Spine* in 1996, for example, found that nearly half the adults in a semitraditional Australian Aboriginal community experienced chronic low-back pain, yet none of them thought of it as a "condition" or as something to complain about it. Instead, they simply lived with it, treating their low-back pain as a normal part of life, like going to the bathroom, and functioning quite well despite it in most cases.

When a different team of researchers did a follow-up study in the same community nearly 20 years later, they found that things had changed—and not for the better. By that time, Western medicine had achieved far greater penetration into the culture, and a majority of those with chronic low-back pain, having received diagnoses and treatment from medical professionals, now explained their pain in the same language of "structural/anatomical vulnerability" that their doctors used. What's more, the individuals in whom these beliefs about pain were most ingrained showed the highest level of dysfunction.

Pain Does Not Require a Diagnosis

The next step in the standard medicalized regime for treating athletic pain is naturally to seek help from a medical professional—either a general practitioner, an orthopedist, a sports medicine specialist, a physical therapist, or a chiropractor, all of whom receive little or no pain science education in their training. The decision to take this step assumes that the athlete is not capable of dealing with the pain on their own, which is a perfectly fair assumption to make when it is already assumed that strong and persistent pain is always an indicator of underlying injury. After all, few athletes own an X-ray machine or an MRI scanner or any of the other fancy technologies that are used to diagnose sports injuries, and just as few possess the credentials or authority to prescribe or administer common treatments, including medication and physical therapy.

The problem with all of this is that it places the athlete in a position of dependency when dealing with pain. It is a proven fact that people in pain feel better and regain function more quickly when they possess a high level of *pain self-efficacy*, which is defined as a belief in one's ability to cope effectively with pain. The medicalization of pain systematically (albeit unintentionally) robs individuals of pain self-efficacy and thereby worsens outcomes. A study led by Kim Bennell of the University of Melbourne and published in *Arthritis Care & Research* in 2015 compared the effects of two different treatment regimens on men and women suffering from knee osteoarthritis. One treatment consisted of a 10-session exercise program, while the second coupled the same exercise program with training in pain-coping skills. Bennell's team saw significantly greater functional improvement in subjects who'd learned pain-coping skills, and one year later, they were still doing better than those who hadn't. The sad irony is that this training in pain-coping skills really did nothing more than counteract the negative impact on pain self-efficacy that is wrought by our current system of treating pain, which seldom includes such training.

So the athlete sees a doctor or physical therapist with little or no education in pain science who endeavors to diagnose the injury and identify its cause. Although the athlete may not be consciously aware of it, a variety of elements of this experience will influence how quickly their pain resolves and they are able to return to full training.

Certain contextual factors are known to improve pain outcomes by positively influencing expectations, while others have the opposite effect. If the doctor actively involves the athlete in understanding their pain and in making treatment decisions, for example, the athlete is more likely to be satisfied with the results. Again, however, this is not the norm. In the typical clinical appointment, the athlete takes a very passive role that further diminishes self-efficacy.

The specific language clinicians employ is another important contextual factor. Have you ever been evaluated by a clinician who used the words *imbalanced*, *weak*, or *tight* to describe parts of your body? Not only are such words usually inaccurate when presented as causes of an athletic injury, but they also stoke a sense of fragility in athletes that is not helpful to long-term prospects for successful pain management.

Pain Does Not Require Treatment

The final step in the standard regime for treating athletic pain is, of course, treatment. There's an old joke that encapsulates what happens all too often at this stage:

> **Doctor:** What seems to be the problem?
> **Patient:** It hurts when I raise my arm.
> **Doctor:** Then don't raise your arm.

It's not a terribly funny joke, and it's even worse advice, yet it's pretty darn close to the advice someone would get from a clinician if they went in complaining of pain around specific movements.

Most athletes are familiar with RICE, a mnemonic that encodes basic guidelines for self-treating musculoskeletal pain. Any guesses on what the first letter stands for? That's right: rest. If it hurts when you run, don't run. If it hurts when you lift weights, don't lift weights. You get the idea.

Now, to be fair to the doctors, it seems like common sense to not do something that hurts. But it turns out that rest is generally not an effective response to musculoskeletal pain, at least not if you intend to use the painful part of your body athletically again. The other letters of the acronym aren't much better. The *I*, for example, stands for ice, and even Gabe Mirkin, the physician who came up with RICE, later admitted that although icing does tend to reduce inflammation, it can also slow the healing process. As for *C*, compression, a 2005 review conducted by Anita Pollard and Gerard Cronin concluded that "little evidence is available to support this kind of treatment." And nine years later, Dutch researchers made a similar judgment on *E*, elevation, reporting that "no evidence based on studies with high levels of evidence is available for the effectiveness of elevation."

The same goes for most other treatments commonly prescribed for athletic pain, including NSAIDs such as ibuprofen. There is no scientific evidence that these medications accelerate the return to full training in athletes whose ability to work out is currently limited by pain, and there's plenty of reason to believe that overreliance on such drugs may delay the return to full training. NSAIDs, in particular, impair soft tissue healing and blunt certain beneficial muscle adaptations to exercise.

OK, if none of the classic pain treatments actually work (and you can toss in fancier treatments, including cupping, lasers, ultrasounds, and dry needling), what *does* work to manage pain, stimulate adaptive tissue remodeling (i.e., healing), and counteract pain's limiting effects on training? Only one treatment can be considered truly essential based on scientific and real-world evidence, and it's pretty much the opposite of what common sense and medical tradition suggest: exercise.

That's right. As strange as it may sound, the closest thing to a panacea for pain associated with movement is movement. Support for this idea comes from an ever-expanding body of research, including a study that was published in the *New England Journal of Medicine* in 2017. Scientists at the University of Copenhagen recruited 50 amateur athletes who were recovering from severe muscle strains and separated them into two groups. Both groups went through a rehabilitation program involving gradually intensifying the use of the injured muscle, but while one group started the program just two days after being injured, the other rested for nine days and then started exercising. All the athletes were tracked until they returned to full participation in their sport. This took an average of 83 days for members of the "rest" group compared to just 62 days for the "exercise" group—a 25 percent difference.

Movement helps athletes who are experiencing pain in a number of ways. On a physiological level, exercise improves function in more or less the same manner it improves fitness, pushing back the limits on what and how much the affected part of the body can do without an unacceptable level of discomfort. At the same time, movement operates on other levels, mitigating pain expectation (hence pain itself), enhancing pain self-efficacy, and more. Add it all up and you're left with one conclusion: The most comprehensive treatment for pain associated with athletic training is training.

If this sounds like a radical concept, well, it is—at least from the perspective of the standard, medicalized process of dealing with athletic pain. As far as most doctors are concerned, training ceases the moment an "injury" (signaled by pain) occurs. But the athletes I work with are always training, whether healthy or hurt. Only the mode of training changes when a problem occurs. An athlete who is able to train the way they want to and is not limited by pain is in training-for-performance mode. If something goes wrong and pain begins to limit an athlete's training to some degree, the athlete switches to what I call Training as Treatment mode. But they're still training.

PAIN IS PERSONAL

You might be questioning my authority to claim that the existing paradigm for helping athletes deal with pain does more harm than good and to suggest that a completely different paradigm is needed. Well, I'm not a doctor, nor am I a scientist. In fact, I'm not even a college graduate! What I am is a lifelong athlete who has made it his professional mission to help other athletes. Hands-on experience has been the primary shaper of my understanding of pain. This is not to say I haven't done my share of reading. However, nothing I learned about pain from books ever jibed with what I knew about pain from working out and playing in the great outdoors. It was a personal encounter with persistent athletic pain that led me to discover a new way of looking at the phenomenon and, ultimately, to assume a leading role in developing and applying a better method of helping athletes work with pain.

Pain Is Shaped by History

When I look back on my journey, it seems as if I was born to do what I'm now doing. I grew up half wild in Hot Springs, Arkansas, a not-quite-town where kids had to make their own fun but where there was plenty of fun to be had if you weren't afraid to take a few risks. It's a miracle that any of us lived to the age of maturity, honestly. I got my first motorcycle when I was in the third grade and promptly set about riding it through the woods at 40 mph. I jumped off roofs, cliffs, and bridges, and I routinely swam 3 miles across Lake Hamilton to get to the Hot Springs Mall. Yet it wasn't until the age of 15 that I hurt myself in any memorable way.

I'd gotten really into martial arts by then—and I mean *really* into them. It all started with weekly lessons in Mahato karate at a local dojo run by a Vietnam veteran who'd learned the method during and after his deployment. To accelerate my progress, I bought all of Bruce Lee's training books and had them bound and laminated, and I even built my own gym around an oak tree on my family's property. It had a climbing ladder, a kickboard, a heavy bag, and a pair of gymnastics rings, all of my own making. I wore the bark off a 20-foot-high branch doing hanging crunches. One day, my buddy John and I were practicing rolls when I landed wrong on my right shoulder and suffered what I would later learn was a third-degree separation.

Sounds painful, right? And it was painful, but no more so than any of a thousand other dings I'd picked up in my reckless youth—at least not initially. What bothered me more was that I couldn't use my arm. John tried to pop the joint into place so we could get back to rolling, but it was a no-go, so I headed up to the house to tell my mom what had happened. As expected, she reacted with annoyance, suggesting (in so many words) that I suck it up. Don't get the wrong idea—my mother cared about my well-being as much as any normal parent. It's just that in my family, a suck-it-up attitude toward pain prevailed—and for good reason, as I will explain in the next chapter.

So it was that instead of whisking me away to the emergency room, as most parents of a 15-year-old boy who came home unable to use his right arm would have done, my folks went out to dinner that evening with friends. Again, in no way did I feel maltreated or neglected by this move. Anything different would have surprised me. But the fact remained that I couldn't use my right arm, and while Mom and Dad enjoyed surf and turf at Mrs. Miller's Chicken & Steakhouse, I lay on the couch trying to figure out what to do. Finding me still on the couch when they returned, my dad resorted to our family's equivalent of whisking me away to the emergency room, which entailed phoning his friend Brian Riley, a thick-necked former rugby player from Boston and the only licensed chiropractor in our area. Brian came over that night, threw me onto a table, angled my lame arm to 45 degrees, braced a foot against the table edge, and yanked away.

I didn't sleep that night. Not a wink. I felt as if I had a migraine in my shoulder, my pulse throbbing deep inside the joint. My primary emotion, though, was not misery or self-pity but amazement. I'd gotten away with so much crazy stuff over the years, and now here I was laid out by a glorified somersault. It made no sense! Still, I trusted I wouldn't be sidelined for very long, and I wasn't. Within a couple of weeks, I was back at the oak tree, climbing the rope ladder, pummeling the heavy bag, and yes, working on my rolls.

Pain Is Shaped by Experience

Despite being severely tested on a routine basis by my next great athletic passion—climbing—the shoulder gave me no more trouble until 2004, when I was 30. The first sign of trouble was a dull ache that I felt not during but between climbing sessions and workouts, which gradually worsened over a period of weeks. I went from being able to do multiple one-arm pull-ups to not even being able to hang from my right arm some days. Like many pain experiences, though, this one ebbed and flowed. I knew I was in for a bad day if it hurt to lift my coffee mug in the morning.

When Thanksgiving rolled around, my wife, Betsy, and I visited her mother at Fort Benning in Georgia. After the holiday, Betsy and I (and Sunshine, our husky-chow mix) packed ourselves inside Butter Bean, our beloved but temperamental '84 Westfalia Vanagon, for the 10-hour drive back to Hot Springs, where we planned to spend the winter with my folks before heading home to Flagstaff. Normally, I would have held Betsy's hand as I drove, but it hurt my shoulder to do so, so I rested my right hand on my lap and steered with my left. Just outside of Winfield, Alabama, we stopped for ice cream, which Betsy spoon-fed to me as we continued along Interstate 22 well after nightfall.

It was then that the red light came on. Every Westfalia owner knows about the dreaded red light that blinks whenever anything goes wrong, which, I hate to admit, is often. Barely five weeks had passed since the last episode, which resulted in a $3,500 motor rebuild that hurt way more than any shoulder injury. Betsy and I had $600 in the bank. At home in Flagstaff, I scraped by as a part-time trainer, part-time barista, and part-time middle school health and wellness teacher. We could ill afford another costly repair.

Nor, however, could I afford to take the risk of pressing ahead with the temperature needle now straying dangerously close to the danger zone. With a heavy sigh, I pulled into the breakdown lane, killed the engine, and popped the top. Within 90 seconds, Betsy and I were in full hangout mode, with our seats rotated toward the rear and our travel-stiffened legs extended.

"What a great car to break down in," Betsy observed.

Before long, a police cruiser pulled up behind us, and I hopped out to chat with the officer. Having explained our situation, I was given the name and number of a place just down the road that offered a towing service. Considering the respectable source of the referral, I was more than a little taken aback when our would-be rescuer turned out to be a scruffy, hoodie-wearing dude in his early 20s who, judging by his mumbling speech and the glazed look in his eyes, was strung out on something potent. Still, it's my nature to give everyone the benefit of the doubt, so I watched in silence as the scruffy dude hooked the winch cable to the van in an incorrect manner that would have resulted in Butter Bean's rear bumper being torn off if I hadn't intervened and gotten her safely mounted.

After a brief detour to a motel to "party," as the dude phrased it, we were delivered unharmed to a surprisingly busy (given the hour) gravel-surfaced complex with a garage, a wrecking yard, the afore-mentioned towing service, and a parts store that doubled as a guns-and-ammo shop. Betsy and I (and Sunshine) slept fitfully in the van as growling wreckers and rumbling semis came and went straight through the night. When I climbed out the next morning, the first thing I saw was a confederate flag magnet lying on the ground at my feet.

I'm not a big believer in omens, but it's hard not to look back on this literal rude awakening as a harbinger of events to come. Westfalias are rare and peculiar vehicles, and not every mechanic knows how to fix them. It didn't take me long to figure out that the mechanic assigned to work on Butter Bean wasn't up to the job. He did far more dismantling under the hood than seemed necessary, contorting the front bumper in the process and looking more and more confounded by the minute. Not wanting to see where all of this was headed, I called the guy who'd rebuilt the motor for me in California.

"Don't let them do anything to your van," he said emphatically.

A bit late for that, I thought. Returning to poor Butter Bean, I told the mechanic to just stop. He did so immediately and with evident relief, then promptly demanded $500 for his work. I blew my stack.

"For what?" I said. "You didn't do anything!"

A heated argument ensued, which I won simply by leaving my wallet right where it belonged, in my back pocket. Our departure was less than triumphant, however. I wish I could say I climbed into Butter Bean, floored the accelerator, and screeched away, showering the useless mechanic with a spray of gravel. As it was, Betsy and I pushed the van across the street to a vacant lot to reassess our situation. Only later did it strike me that my shoulder, which the day before had hurt when I tried to hold Betsy's hand, didn't trouble me in the slightest as I played tugboat with the one-and-a-half-ton vehicle, and it was later still that I learned the likely reason: My expectation of pain was thwarted by a displacement of my attentional focus. In other words, my shoulder didn't hurt when I pushed the van because I was much more concerned about our present predicament than I was about my shoulder.

At the second garage, I tried bleeding the coolant system in the hope that doing so would at least allow us to escape by sundown, which was fast approaching. We were within sight of the B and B where Betsy had made a reservation when the van overheated a second time, and we were just barely able to coast the remaining distance.

In the morning, I made some calls and found a U-Haul dealer 20 miles away. Our plan was to hitchhike there, rent a truck and a trailer, and drag Butter Bean the rest of the way to Hot Springs. Our thumbs were ignored, however, and we ended up completing the journey through a mix of walking and running, arriving only to discover we were in the wrong location. I dialed the same phone number I'd dialed previously and was informed that the place I'd meant to go was just closing.

"Wait for us!" I pleaded, already beginning to run. "We'll be right there."

No sooner was this ordeal behind us than my shoulder pain came back. Years would pass before I discovered what was really going on, but from my present perspective, it couldn't be more obvious. I think of myself as a cheerful person, but this was not the most cheerful season of my life. There was the difficult reality of Betsy's and my lean financial circumstances. But these were by no means my only concern. My first marriage had ended 18 months earlier, and I hadn't fully processed the emotional trauma. Also, one of the reasons Betsy and I had chosen to spend the winter in Hot Springs was that the South has a lot of great undiscovered venues for bouldering, but it rained almost constantly that winter, so we got very little climbing done. To earn my keep, I went to work digging postholes on the family horse farm. It's honest work, the same work I'd done when I was 13, but doing it again at 30 seemed symbolic of a life that hadn't gone very far. And to top it all off, I couldn't help but worry that the return of my boyhood shoulder pain was an indication that my peak climbing years were coming to an end—or worse, that they were already behind me.

It never even crossed my mind at the time that these factors might be contributing to my discomfort. Instead, like any other athlete, I assumed my pain indicated an injury. But subsequent testing by multiple specialists back in Flagstaff revealed no significant underlying structural damage. The shoulder sure felt broken, but it wasn't. The true underlying cause of my pain, I now believe, was my memory of separating the same shoulder as a teenager, which made it a likely location for future pain to manifest in response to the physical stress imposed on it by training and climbing. My passion for climbing added an element of hypervigilance and overprotection that sensitized me to trouble in that critically needed part of my body. And the final piece was the cumulative *allostatic load* (stress) of this period of my life. All that stress had to come out somehow, and in retrospect, it's no surprise that it came out in the form of pain in my right shoulder.

Eventually, the pain went away, as athletic pain almost always does if the person experiencing it doesn't give up. Indeed, it wasn't anything specific beyond not giving up that brought me through the ordeal. Resting, which I tried more than once, didn't help. On the other hand, neither did forcing myself to train as if the pain didn't exist. Nor did the various doctors, physical therapists, and chiropractors I consulted, except for one who brought about some improvement in my condition not because of anything specific he did with me but because of my confidence in him. What *did* help, in the end, was my own self-guided process of learning to work around and through my limitations until they disappeared. I know that sounds rather vague, but in the 15-plus years since I got my shoulder back, I have figured out how to make this process both systematic and replicable, and by the time you finish reading this book, you will be fully capable of applying it in your training.

A NEW WAY TO PROCESS PAIN

By no means have I done it alone. In fact, I wouldn't have done it at all had I not discovered the biopsychosocial model of pain and the small but growing community of fellow coaches and clinicians who base their practices on it. This discovery came about quite by accident, like finding the Fountain of Youth when you were merely looking for lost treasure. I emerged from my long and frustrating second bout of shoulder pain with a determination to do whatever I could to spare other athletes from having to go through a similar experience. Still in the thrall of the structural model of athletic pain, I embarked on a misguided quest to learn everything there was to know about *functional anatomy*, or how muscles and joints function, and *pathoanatomy*, or how muscles and joints occasionally "malfunction," so I could stop these structures from failing to work properly (thereby causing pain) and get them working again in those cases where I got involved too late to play a preventive role.

This ambition relied on a false assumption that there are neatly defined right and wrong ways for the body to move and that pain and injury are caused by wrong movements. In my defense, this was (and is) the prevailing view of strength and conditioning specialists, physical therapists, sports medicine doctors, and other experts, including those I most trusted. And where did the experts get this notion? Well, from science, supposedly.

Only when I took a deep dive into pain science—not just reading studies but attending conferences that only folks with advanced degrees were supposed to attend, joining professional online discussion groups that I had no business being admitted to, and so forth—did I discover the evidence simply does not support the structural model by which many pain experiences are explained. From there, one final step led me to the biopsychosocial model that now serves as the foundation of my efforts to help athletes manage pain.

Aside from my beliefs about pain, another thing that has changed is my attitude. I used to think I had it all figured out, or at least that I was close to having all the right answers, but I now recognize that I don't know everything and never will. My current approach to helping athletes is collaborative, more focused on asking questions than on reciting stock answers. I no longer try to "fix" my clients' problems;

instead, I work with them to discover solutions that are seldom perfect. It's a much less certain process than my old way of doing things, but it's also far more effective.

Having been on this path for a while now, I've developed a reputation as a sort of pain whisperer. As such, I see a lot of last-chancers at my gym in Flagstaff—athletes who have exhausted the traditional methods without success and are desperate enough to gamble on a different approach to musculoskeletal care. A good example is Ann, an accomplished poet and avid hiker and backpacker who came to me at age 73 complaining of persistent back pain—in fact, she was scheduled for spinal fusion surgery. As I do with all my clients, I handed Ann a pad and pen to take notes with (my way of getting clients actively involved in the process from the outset) and sat down with her for an initial consultation that concluded with my saying, in so many words, "OK, let's try some stuff and figure this out together."

The stuff we tried consisted almost entirely of exercise, of course, and it worked. Ann ended up canceling her surgery, and years later, at age 78, she was almost able to complete a full unassisted pull-up. Today, whenever her friends complain to her of knee pain and the like, she tells them, "You should exercise!"

Ann is just one of many clients—young and old, weekend warrior and elite—whom I've had the honor of helping through the Training as Treatment approach to managing athletic pain. There are others, I confess, that I have not been able to help as much as I wanted to. Any clinician who paints themselves as a miracle worker and either boasts of or implies a 100 percent success rate is not to be trusted, and I want you to trust me.

To that end, I'm going to proceed along a different path than the one you might be accustomed to from reading other training guides. I've told you a little about my personal story, but I'm going to tell you a good deal more in the next few chapters—not because I'm so interesting but because pain is personal, hence a more personal approach is likely the best way to help you fully understand and embrace the new science of pain and my Training as Treatment principles. Both are completely unfamiliar to most athletes and are also counterintuitive in many respects. Allowing you to see how I came to understand and embrace these things will, I hope, better serve my goal of persuading you that my methodology is worth a try.

The larger purpose of this book is to teach you everything you need to know to practice the Training as Treatment method in your own athletic endeavors, and this is the job of the second half. In Chapter 6, we'll delve into the new science of athletic pain and injury, which is kind of mind-blowing once you understand it. From there, we'll move on to discuss the various allostatic contributors to pain and how to manage them, and we'll also go over pain self-efficacy and the concrete steps you can take to make pain your employee rather than your employer. Then we'll hit the gym, where we'll learn important concepts such as *descending analgesia* and *symptom modification* and specific exercises and processes that, through these and other mechanisms, treat pain more effectively than traditional means. We'll then wrap things up with a discussion of several commonly diagnosed injuries that aren't really injuries and some guidelines on how to find and identify coaches, doctors, and therapists who can aid versus hinder your efforts at pain management.

Let's be clear: I'm not here to *cure* your pain. As I stated at the outset, pain is an unavoidable part of life and of the athletic experience especially. What I *am* here to do is permanently transform your relationship with pain. I don't care particularly which facts or techniques in this book you still retain five years from now. All I care about is that your new relationship with pain is one where you understand it better, feel a greater sense of control, and are less limited by it. And I truly do care. My sincere personal investment in helping you, combined with my experience and hard-won knowledge, is what I bring to our partnership. All I need from you are a shared goal and an open mind.

2

GET BACK ON THE HORSE

You'd be hard-pressed to find a more painful profession than that of horse jockey. There may be more dangerous jobs out there, but I doubt there's one that hurts as much. The average career for a jockey lasts about nine months. My dad raced horses for nearly 37 years, and he was still riding thoroughbreds—albeit no longer competitively—at 72, when he was found unconscious on the track at Louisiana Downs in Shreveport, Louisiana, his horse wandering alone some distance away. So lifeless did he appear that no particular rush was made to summon medical aid, and though he did survive, the traumatic brain injury he suffered that day affects him even now.

It's a miracle my father didn't sooner suffer an injury he would never fully recover from. By the time he turned seven, he'd broken his right arm so many times in cotton-patch racing accidents that after yet another fall, there was some discussion about amputating it. When I picture my father as I first knew him, I see purple hoof-prints marking the skin of his wiry 5-foot-4-inch body. To be clear, this is not an image from a single incident but rather a composite memory of numerous trampling episodes. Dad broke his neck on two occasions and had his jaw wired shut a couple of times as well.

For a period of time, a hospital bed sat in the middle of our living room, ready when needed, which was often. One accident left him with no pulse—dead on the track for several minutes.

It takes a special kind of person to race horses for three and a half decades, and David Earl Whited is one of a kind. Born in Odessa, Texas, in 1948, he inherited Native American blood from his mother, a full-blooded Choctaw, and (how do I say this?) grifter blood from his father. All joking aside, I loved Papa, as I called my grandfather, but he was a horse trader both literally and figuratively. Before Dad was old enough to read, Papa had him stealing moonshine at night and abetting various other forms of mischief. From there he graduated to racing horses against grown men, breaking bones as routinely as other kids his age lost baby teeth.

At 13, my father-to-be decided he'd had enough. One winter's morning, he snuck away from the house (not difficult, as he was loosely supervised) and made his way to the westbound side of Interstate 20, where he put a thumb out. A few days later, he landed in Phoenix, arriving just in time for the seasonal opening of Sunland Park, the local horse track. He found work there and was soon fully immersed in the curious world of horse racing and again breaking bones. According to family lore, Dad was confined to bed for an extended period after a particularly brutal fall, except it wasn't a bed but a wooden box. He survived on a ration of one hamburger a day, which was brought to him by a kindhearted fellow trainer. It was like something out of a Dickens novel.

Given his experience with horses, his indifference to pain, and his limited options, Dad was all but destined to become a professional jockey. But he truly liked it. Everything about the lifestyle appealed to him: the sketchiness, the itinerancy, the excitement, the risk. It was a lot like joining the circus, another lurid subculture peopled by oddballs and misfits roaming from place to place in a perpetual quest for the big score. He called it a destination addiction.

Horse-racing season varies geographically, shifting from location to location every couple of months, and young David quickly fell into a rhythm of hopscotching between Louisville and New Orleans and Atlantic City and other racing hotbeds as the season unfolded. On a stop in El Paso in 1996, he met Bonnie Charleen Clatfelter, the local rodeo queen and my future mom. Famously cocksure on the racing circuit ("Who's racing for second?" he was known to taunt his fellow jockeys at the starting gate), Dad wasn't shy about showing his interest in El Paso's most eligible bachelorette. Strikingly handsome, with sharp southern Native American features and a bronze complexion, he couldn't fail to make an impression. But Mom didn't go for over-confident guys, and Dad had to work for her attention, eventually succeeding through the time-tested method of showing off his dance moves at Cattleman's Steakhouse, a venue that still stands today.

The couple settled down in Hot Springs, Arkansas, another horse-racing hotbed, though the phrase *settled down* is hardly accurate in this case. I like to say I was raised on the front floorboards and rear dog shelves of a series of cash-bought Cadillacs, rolling from track to track with Dad behind the wheel, Mom beside him, my older brother David Jr. sprawled across the back seat, and a U-Haul trailer swaying behind. The gentle friction between tire rubber and asphalt lulled me to sleep at night. I still remember the faint smell of new plastic on those carpets. Six times a year, year in and year out, we left behind whichever trailer or motel we'd called home for the past eight weeks and moved on to the next one.

It was no way to raise a family, needless to say, as became clear one night in Atlantic City. My mom and David and I were huddled up inside a room at a seedy off-brand motel in a dodgy part of town while Dad raced when some desperate soul tried to break in. Not one to cower in closets in such situations, Mom was able to scare away the would-be intruder, but on learning of the episode, Dad decided he wasn't going to take any more chances, so he bought a special lock that we used to protect ourselves during future stays in dangerous places. Only in hindsight do I recognize the pitifulness of the comfort that lock gave me.

Around the time I entered third grade, our family made a long-overdue transition to something more closely resembling a normal home life. Even then, my childhood remained far from mundane. It was like being the son of Evel Knievel, the cape-wearing motorcycle daredevil of the 1970s whose movies we owned and watched repeatedly in reel-to-reel format. Any normal adrenaline junkie would have gotten thrills enough from falling off horses, but Dad supplemented these contretemps with extracurricular stunts such as attempting to jump over 20 watermelons on a motorcycle. Had it been 15 watermelons, he'd have stood a chance, but as it was, he came up short, landing on his face and coming away with a scar that remains visible on his right temple.

Alas, adrenaline wasn't his only craving. Dad's failed watermelon stunt took place on a small island where his primary attraction was a liquor store to which he paid almost daily visits to replenish his ever-vanishing supply of Jameson's. At home, the playroom my brother and I shared doubled as a bar, complete with saloon doors, a pool table, and whiskey rails. Our father's beer of choice was Coors, which was hard to find back then, so he did the logical thing and bought an entire pallet and had it trucked out from Colorado.

Clearly, he had a problem. But he also had a big heart, and he loved his wife and children more than anything, so when Mom delivered an ultimatum after an ugly scene one night—I believe her exact words were *Tonight's the night you pick drinking or your family*—Dad quit cold turkey and, as far as I know, never relapsed. It must have been hard for him, but he made it look easy, as was his way.

One thing that did not change as we put down roots in Hot Springs was the centrality of horses to our daily existence. Dad transformed our property into a full-service thoroughbred training center, creating a state-of-the-art three-quarter-mile training track surfaced in the precise ratio of silt, sand, and clay trainers preferred; constructing a horse barn out of materials from a Kroger grocery store he purchased and subsequently demolished in Louisiana; and cobbling together various other amenities, including a public kitchen. Word got out, and horse trainers soon came flocking with their equine athletes, creating a tremendous advantage for my father in the ruthlessly competitive racing game, where jockeys are constantly angling to identify and score the choicest mounts and trainers are continually scouting out the hottest jockeys for their horses.

It's difficult to overstate the tenuousness of the horse jockey's professional and financial positions. Securing mounts is only half the battle. In the so-called sport of kings, there are no finisher medals. Riders receive a pittance for merely participating in races—not nearly enough to survive on. The real money comes from winning, placing, and showing—just as it does for the bettors, who are the wellspring of everyone's increase—and even the best jockeys have scarcely more control over an outcome than gamblers. Truly, my dad was one of the best, winning 3,790 races in his career and earning enshrinement in the horse-racing hall of fame. Every once in a while, though, Dad would have a run of bad luck, riding a series of horses that, for whatever reason, performed poorly, causing trainers to sour on him for a period. Sudden austerity measures (such as our cash-purchased Cadillacs being sold cheap) were always a sign that he'd hit one of these fallow periods.

Dad often spoke of the Big Horse, a mythical supersteed that never spooked, got hurt, or had a bad outing and always won, single-hoofedly purging all the uncertainty from our precarious existence. I'm not sure how the whole thing got started, but over the years, the Big Horse became an important, if fanciful, figure in the Whited clan. When we conjured him up, which was often, we always did so half-jokingly, but as we all know, half-joking is also half-serious. I, for one, certainly hoped the Big Horse would turn up one day.

The subtext of much of our obsessive horse talk was health. To have any chance of finishing in the money, Dad had to compete, and to compete, both he and the horse he rode in on had to be healthy—or at least healthy enough. He fussed over horses in much the same way multibillion-dollar professional sports teams' support staffs (including doctors, trainers, massage therapists, and nutritionists) fuss over their players. Racehorses are bona fide athletes, after all, and like other athletes, they are always walking a fine line between peak fitness and some form of dreaded injury, such as shin bucking. My dad was not a worrier by nature, but to the extent he did worry, it was invariably about the condition of the horses he rode or might ride, and a measure of this concern trickled down to me. My peers knew how to level up in video games; I knew how to palpate a horse's fetlocks for inflammation.

Dad gave just as much attention to his own health, but he was less vocal about it. When he got injured and couldn't ride, we might hear him complain about the lost income, but we never heard a peep about the pain he experienced. And pain alone certainly never stopped him from riding—for this to happen, he needed to be injured to the point of being physically incapable of performing. That old exhortation "Get back on the horse that bucked you" was Dad's modus operandi. He rode through just about every kind of injury imaginable, including broken legs and a broken back. One time, his boot got caught in the starting gate at the beginning of a race, a freakish mishap that left his foot a gory mess inside the boot's mangled leather. Recognizing that even if he succeeded in extricating his foot from the boot to receive first aid, he'd probably be unable to stuff it back in, he instead MacGyvered the situation with duct tape and finished out the day's racing.

I don't mean to give the impression that David Whited was a macho man bent on proving his toughness to others. As a matter of fact, in his mind, pain was just part of the job. He dealt with it quietly not because he believed in some archaic code of manhood but rather because dealing with it was necessary and talking about it served no purpose. The thought of making his pain someone else's problem, of delegating the responsibility of fixing it, never occurred to him. Only in the most extreme scenarios would he seek medical attention, and even then he often overruled the doctors, like the time he received an unwanted leg cast and sawed it off as soon as he got home. As fatigue is to the marathon runner, so was pain to my father: something he had to work through himself to achieve his goals.

In this regard, Dad was representative of a bygone time, an example of how people handled pain before it became medicalized. In the preceding chapter, I described a pair of studies involving an Aboriginal community in Australia, the first of which found that although low-back pain was common among its members, they did not think of it as a condition per se, and they almost never spoke of it. It's my belief that their reason for keeping silent on the subject was essentially the same as Dad's reason for not bringing up the topic of pain associated with his many racing injuries. They likely saw no reason to present it to one another as a problem. It would have been like complaining of being sleepy every single night just before bedtime. Why make a big to-do out of a normal and natural feeling that one can easily manage for oneself?

Nowadays, medical professionals apply novel terms like *desensitization* and *graded exposure* to the pain-management methods that folks like my dad used to practice as a matter of course. Dad was particularly adept at what is today referred to as *symptom modification*, figuring out various ways to adjust his riding style when pain prevented him from riding in the usual way.

MY OWN EDUCATION IN SELF-RELIANCE

The course of my life was profoundly influenced by my early exposure to my father's approach to pain management, yet I did not recognize this for myself until relatively recently—and even then, only with outside help. I was with a client dealing with running-related hip discomfort, and in an effort to normalize and show empathy for her pain experience, I shared an anecdote about my father, to which she responded with the unexpected words "Well, that explains a few things." She meant, of course, that my having borne witness to episodes like the one I'd just described at an impressionable age explained my interest in pain and injury, my deep-seated desire to help athletes, and my pragmatic approach to managing pain—all of which, I now see, I got either directly or indirectly from my family's peculiar relationship to pain and injury.

There was a time—very brief—when I even toyed with the idea of becoming a jockey myself. It made sense, kind of. I loved horses, I enjoyed risk-taking, I had a willing mentor, and I was a runt. Dad knew better than to actively encourage me to take up the family business—a step that certainly would have elicited a second ultimatum from my mother—but he did find ways to nudge me in the direction he wanted, much as he did with horses, by making them think they were making their own decisions. In the summer between my freshman and sophomore years of high school, Dad put me to work on the farm, where one thing led to another, and before I knew it, I was working horses, rising before dawn to ride thoroughbreds at fantastic speeds around a freshly groomed track. I loved it, and I might have gone further down this path by my own initiative if I hadn't undergone a significant growth spurt that put the whole fantasy to bed.

The same sudden jump in bodily proportions that killed my jockeying prospects had the opposite effect on my other sporting outlets of football and track-and-field. I was your classic fastest-kid-on-the-block type, able to count on one hand the number of times I'd lost a 100-meter race since my first youth track meets in elementary school. In the football-crazy South, there was no way for a boy with my kind of speed to avoid the gridiron, and though I had zero interest in football, I went with the flow and joined the Lake Hamilton Wolves as a seventh grader.

The experience was a mixed bag for me. While I chafed at the constraints of team play, I did like my coach. A former Mr. Arkansas bodybuilder who'd since grown as big as a refrigerator, Coach MacIntosh trained us like soldiers—and I mean that almost literally. He barked at us as if he were auditioning for the role of a foulmouthed, masochistic drill sergeant in a war movie, sweat flying off his handlebar mustache, cheeks purpling, neck tendons popping out. He was in possession of a wooden paddle with holes drilled into it so he could swing it at our backsides with less air resistance, hence greater velocity. Among the other 12-year-olds he subjected to such histrionics was my buddy Adam Brown, who remains to this day—more than a decade after he died heroically on a battlefield in Afghanistan—the toughest human being I have ever known. In 1999, when Adam returned to Arkansas from California after earning a Navy SEAL trident, I asked him how hard the infamous six-month BUD/S training program was, and his blasé answer—"Really hard"—failed to satisfy my curiosity.

"Harder than Coach MacIntosh's practices?" I pressed.

"About the same," he deadpanned.

Bleeding, projectile vomiting, and losing consciousness were routine occurrences in those practices. Adam and I loved them because of how much we suffered. In fact, I enjoyed testing my physical and mental limits in Tuesday conditioning drills far more than I enjoyed playing to win in Saturday games, what with all the absurd hoopla surrounding those gladiatorial spectacles. There are some folks in this world who, for whatever reason, get their kicks from seeing how much they can take and how far they can go, and in early adolescence, I discovered I was one of them.

The following summer, I left home for Camp Kanakuk, a youth athletic camp held near Branson, Missouri, just over the Arkansas border. Coach MacIntosh wasn't there (most of the counselors were college athletes), but the same no-pain-no-gain culture prevailed. The facility's weight room resembled a medieval torture chamber: a dark, dank, dirt-walled concrete slab upon which teenage boys grunted and screamed under the burden of loads of rusty metal. Recently, I caught myself telling someone I threw up daily at Camp Kanakuk, but that's an exaggeration. A very slight exaggeration.

Whereas most of my fellow first timers found themselves being pushed to extremes of exertion previously unimagined, I was in familiar territory, having pushed myself just as hard back home, where for kicks, I did things like jerry-rig my own weight sled and harness and sprint across the front yard like a rabid mule towing a tipped-over minivan. I liked to invent new exercises, seeing no reason a 12-year-old farm boy shouldn't do so. The one that comes to mind is an insanely risky stunt where I hung upside down from a tree branch and contracted my hamstrings and hip flexors, causing my body to swing up like that of an Olympic diver doing a swan dive. Kids: Do not try this at home!

My instincts told me that in the pursuit of greater fitness and performance, I needed to be self-reliant—to chase progress by playing around, trying stuff out, testing hunches, creatively working around obstacles, and learning by doing. This process was steered by the guardrails of fatigue, effort tolerance, and yes, pain, which revealed my limits and, in so doing, guided my progress, sort of like how a hand on a wall guides one down a darkened hallway. Unfortunately, future miseducation would teach me to see pain as different from these other constraints, but as a kid, that was not the case. I twisted ankles, bruised bones, strained muscles, and woke up sore, but I dealt with these matters the same way I dealt with projectile vomiting or losing a sprint or struggling to complete a rep: by mixing things up, trying stuff out, and keeping at it until I was able to do more.

I find it rather telling that the one time I broke from my habit of self-managing pain during my school years and sought help from a clinician, it did not turn out well for me. In the middle of my first season of high school football, I developed persistent pain in my right hip. When I mentioned it to my coach, he suggested I go in for X-rays, so I did. The images revealed what was described to me as a slipped growth plate in the hip joint. Visibly concerned, the doctor warned me that if the problem wasn't "fixed" (his exact word choice), I risked losing not only my ability to clock 4.5 seconds in the 40-yard dash but also my ability to walk normally. He prescribed a round of chiropractic adjustments to get the plate back in place and urged me to avoid stressing the hip in the meantime.

If I had known then what I know now—namely, that words like "fixed" and other kinds of catastrophizing language negatively impact expectations and worsen outcomes—I would have disregarded my coach's advice to get X-rays and addressed the pain with the usual measures of working around and toward the sensation as it permitted, and I'd have been better off. Instead, I developed a fear of pain and "stressing the hip" that bothered me even more than the pain itself. Still, the pain diminished and ultimately vanished as I gradually lost faith in my doctor's opinion and went back to doing things my way. Alas, I would require a few more lessons like this one before I made a conscious commitment to doing things my way once and for all—not only for myself but also for the athletes I serve.

But back to Camp Kanakuk. On a handful of occasions during the steamy, mosquito-plagued fortnight I spent there, we all trooped off to nearby locations for various activities. On one such occasion, our destination was Hemmed-in-Hollow Falls, and the activity was rappelling. We received a quick lesson peppered with the usual warnings and admonitions, harnessed up, and bounded down a bluff that, according to Google, was 209 feet in height but seemed twice that at the time. At the bottom, we were invited to climb back to the top, an invitation that only one camper accepted: me.

We've all had the experience of trying something for the first time and discovering that it felt intensely, inexplicably right, so right that we knew instantly we wanted to do it again and again and eventually master it. No sooner had my fingers found purchase on the rock face and my feet left the ground than the whole world vanished. Nothing remained but the cliff, my body, and my total absorption in the task of reaching the top. I remember thinking—not thinking, *feeling*—*This is where I belong.* It was a feeling I'd never experienced before, not even in martial arts. Physical conditioning came close, as it was something I wished to keep doing and eventually master, but climbing spoke to my very soul.

That feeling ended all too soon, however, and without any real prospect for a reprise. When I tried to tell my friends back home in Hot Springs about the experience, they received my words with blank stares, either having no idea what I was talking about or mistakenly thinking I was referring to mountain climbing. And if I specified rock climbing, it was clear from their now-baffled looks that they were picturing me monkeying around on a rock pile. Rock climbing was literally unheard of in Arkansas in the 1980s. I might as well have been describing a surfing trip to Siberians. When I started climbing regularly a few years later, I routinely ascended local features that no one had ever climbed before. *Because no one had ever thought of it.*

In the meantime, I satisfied my climbing yen as best I could vicariously by subscribing to and devouring magazines like *Backpacker* and *Outside*. When I was 16, *Backpacker* ran a feature on the San Juan Mountains in Colorado that had a galvanizing effect on me. It so happened that around that same time, I experienced my first automobile accident. I was on my way to school, behind the wheel of an old secondhand Celica my folks bought for me, when I came upon a familiar vehicle that belonged to a classmate of mine and was being driven at a comically slow rate of speed (because, I would later learn, she didn't know how to shift out of second gear). The road was quite narrow, but I had just enough room to get around her, so I began to pass. Just then, my classmate swerved left to avoid a dead raccoon, sending the Celica into a culvert, which in turn ramped the vehicle straight into a telephone pole. Thanks to my seat belt, I wasn't hurt, but the car was totaled, so I had no wheels for the road trip I was fixing to make to Colorado for spring break with my buddy John (the same John who tried to pop my shoulder back into place after that ill-fated karate roll a few years earlier).

The fate of the proposed adventure now rested on my ability to gain my dad's permission to borrow his beloved truck, a long-bed Ford with a horn that played Dixie. He used it almost daily for bailing hay and other farm chores. I didn't like my chances, but as luck would have it, he happened to not need the vehicle during the week I wanted it, and I got the keys.

John and I drove into the wee hours of the first night, making it across the Colorado border before stopping to sleep in the long bed, which still smelled of hay. The second leg of our journey brought us to Yankee Boy Basin, where we camped between day-long peak-bagging excursions, summitting several fourteeners, including Mount Sneffels (14,158 feet) and Wilson Peak (14,016 feet). The happiness I felt throughout that magical week of freedom cannot be overstated. For the second time in my young life—the first time since being on the cliff face at Hemmed-in-Hollow Falls—I had a sense of belonging right where I was. I knew in my bones that one way or another, my future needed to contain a lot more of this.

I dreaded the return to my fish-out-of-water existence in Hot Springs, Arkansas, as intensely as a condemned man dreads sunrise. Every town in America has disaffected teens who can't wait to get the hell out, and I very much fit this stereotype. I loved exercise and sport but not in the all-encompassing way my teammates did, or were expected to, and the aspects I did enjoy—running and lifting weights and challenging my personal limits—came with too many other things, such as hard partying and extracurricular violence, that seemed endemic to the southern football culture, further fueling my disillusionment with traditional sports. My less-than-all-in attitude toward being a member of the Lake Hamilton varsity football team did not escape the notice of our coach, and after three seasons as its starting tailback, 1 was kicked off the team in my junior year. And although 1 loved learning and 1 knew 1 was smart—diving deep into subjects ranging from Eastern philosophy to exercise physiology in my own time—1 did not enjoy school, nor did 1 do particularly well. In fact, 1 barely graduated, squeaking by with a mix of Cs and Ds.

RYAN WHITED, PERSONAL TRAINER

Given all of this, you might expect that 1 would have caught the first train out after receiving my diploma, but the reality is that my sudden freedom paralyzed me and 1 struggled to choose a direction. After an ill-conceived and very brief college stint in Texas, 1 decided to become a personal trainer. 1 researched the various certification options (the sheer number of which cast a subtle taint on the whole lot of them) and settled on the National Federation of Personal Trainers because it was cheap and quick. 1 sent away for a study kit, studied, took the certification exam at the nearest testing center, and was notified by mail a couple of weeks later that I'd passed.

Back then, just about anyone with a pulse and a certification could get a job at a big-box gym—it's the same today, actually—and 1 soon got one in Hot Springs. On my third or fourth day, 1 had an experience that set the tone for my fraught relationship with the fitness training and physical therapy establishments going forward. My client that day was an overweight young man of about my own age. As part of the gym's standard onboarding procedure, 1 was required to use a pair of fat calipers to estimate his body fat level. Even at 21, 1 knew it was a sham. Not only did the calipers yield notoriously inaccurate results that differed wildly from those generated by the gold-standard method of the time (hydrostatic weighing), but they also yielded inconsistent results. Even an experienced user of the instrument would likely get three different body fat estimates if they took measurements from the same individual three times consecutively.

Worse than these flaws, though, was how the measuring procedure made my client *feel*, as I could clearly tell from his body language. Heck, the poor guy already knew he was overweight—that's the reason he'd hired me! And here I was, squeezing his fat rolls with a set of plastic pinchers that seemed designed to humiliate. I would even go so far as to characterize the procedure's effect as dehumanizing. It made my client feel like a *thing*, a helpless object that I, the omniscient expert, would make better by working on it. Naive as I was still in many ways, I understood that the asymmetrical power dynamics established by the caliper charade were the opposite of helpful, and I vowed privately never to use those stupid things again. And I didn't.

Trouble was, fat calipers weren't the only sham device for measuring health and fitness parameters, and as much as I hate to admit it, there were a few I later bought into. Among these was the goniometer, a tool that physical therapists use to measure joint range of motion. Imagine the love child of a ruler and a draftsman's compass and you'll have a pretty good idea of what a goniometer looks like. While it looks scientific, it is a product of pure pseudoscience, serving no purpose other than to lead athletes to think they *need* a physical therapist to fix what's wrong with them and fostering a state of dependence where the athlete sees themselves as unable to manage their pain on their own.

Like fat calipers, goniometers are woefully imprecise. An experienced physical therapist can measure joint range of motion just as (in)accurately by eyeballing it. Even if they were reliable, though, goniometers don't help athletes any more than fat calipers help personal training clients. In fact, they do more harm than good by promoting a bogus pathoanatomical understanding of pain that roots an athlete's pain experience in flawed movement patterns that are, in turn, rooted in structural imbalances. They're Exhibit A in my indictment of the medicalization of pain—a well-meant but utterly misguided process that has stripped athletes of their power to self-manage pain and turned them into patients.

Don't get me wrong; I believe that science has much to contribute to pain management. Today, I try to base my own clinical practices on empirical evidence whenever possible. But science is a social institution like any other, and as such, it is not without flaws. One of those flaws is a certain kind of arrogance. Science tends to be dismissive of things like intuition, folk practices, and atheoretical trial-and-error problem-solving. Scientists and trained clinicians are often biased toward tools that seem scientific (such as fat calipers and goniometers) while, at the same time, carrying an unrecognized prejudice against brute coping methods such as my dad's choice to duct-tape his foot and boot together so he could get back on the horse and feed his family.

I'm not suggesting my dad had pain management all figured out or that in taking after him, I am on a path of total enlightenment. But I do believe our method of accepting pain as normal is superior to anything espoused by the medical establishment prior to the advent of the biopsychosocial model. An athlete's best approach to pain management is one where science complements and augments the self-management methodology that once existed everywhere and that my father apotheosized. Championing this approach has become my life's work, but it was a long road that brought me here.

LEARN BY DOING

At the eastern edge of the Ouachita Mountains, 8 or 9 miles from the old Whited family farm in Hot Springs, Arkansas, stands an outcropping of novaculite—a chert-like rock found nowhere else on earth—that in my early adult years became a refuge to which I retreated at every opportunity. A place to be alone with my thoughts. A place to immerse myself in the beauty of nature. And a place to push my physical limits.

If you were to visit this site today, hike the very steep hillside, and scrape away the dead leaves carpeting the loose rock underneath with the toe of a boot, you would find a narrow rut, clearly man-made, tracing a line from the bottom to the top. The man who made that rut was me, with my own two feet, by running up the hillside as hard as I could over and over and over again. It took about five minutes to reach the first escarpment, the marker I had chosen for my finish line, and another five minutes to catch my breath. A witness to these exertions would have assumed I was either training for something or insane, and well, I wasn't training for anything.

The kind of person who would sprint up a mountainside repeatedly for no particular reason is also the kind of person who, wanting desperately to rock climb but lacking the proper equipment, would climb anyway. The expensive climbing shoes I saw in magazines looked to me a lot like the cheap aqua socks I owned already, so I climbed in aqua socks and learned the hard way just how misleading appearances can be. The hard, sticky rubber of a climbing shoe is not at all like the sole of an aqua sock. On another occasion, I was soloing a small cliff, perhaps 40 feet in height, when I began to lose my grip (literally, I mean). Having noted a well-positioned pine tree before making the ascent, I made a split-second decision to kick away from the bluff and wrap the trunk in a lifesaving bear hug.

I got my first real climbing gear as a gift from my parents on Christmas Day, 1994. Not knowing just how woefully inadequate the kit was for the uses I had in mind for it, I took it straight to my little sanctuary to test it out on an 80-foot cliff that was the site's major climbing feature. My first mistake was using a bent-gate carabiner to clip my harness to the rope, unaware that this type of carabiner was not intended for such applications because it has the propensity to pop open. My second mistake was recruiting my buddy Adam to serve as my belayer. Since our football days, Adam had gotten hooked on meth and was a few years away from transforming himself into a war hero. Despite his struggles, he remained one of my closest friends and my go-to wingman for misadventure, so I had no hesitation in putting my life in his hands, almost literally, in this ill-fated undertaking.

The cliff topped out with a 20-degree overhang, the trickiest part of the climb. Despite my poor choices in equipment and human assistance, I made it all the way up without incident and secured an anchor that would bear my weight so I could be lowered back down to terra firma. Hanging from one arm, my fingertips tensed, I called down to Adam to lower me. About a millisecond before I let go, I heard a click and saw the rope end that was supposed to be attached to my harness swing away from me. I froze in disbelief, my heart thundering with the understanding I'd come as close to dying as a person could without sustaining a scratch. Willing myself calm, I reached out and snagged the rope with my left hand as it swung back toward me, reclipped the carabiner to my harness, and began my descent, trying not to think about what had almost happened.

The next day, I embarked on a mission to fully educate myself about climbing—purchasing, reading, and rereading every credible climbing book in print, which wasn't as onerous as it might sound because there were only a handful of such books in existence then. The newest and best of these was authored by John "Verm" Sherman, creator of the V scale of bouldering difficulty. Considered the bible of the sport, *Stone Crusade* featured an engrossing mix of vivid personality profiles and gorgeous photography that inspired my shift from rope climbing to bouldering.

As I look back on this formative stage of my climbing journey, I am struck by how very much in keeping it was with my overall approach to sport (and life). I learn by doing, and sometimes—often, in fact—I leap before I look. While I recognize the value of absorbing the wisdom of those who know more than I do, for me, the "doing" part always comes first. While I can't deny that my learning style can be both high-risk and occasionally high-consequence, I wouldn't have it any other way because the other way—studying first and then doing—is artificially limiting not just for me but for any athlete.

To be honest, school was never my jam. It's not that I don't like to read—I love to read—I just prefer to design my own curricula and go at my own pace. Experiential learning has remained a dependable strategy for me through the years, a faithful tool that can be used for a multitude of applications and rarely lets me down, even with respect to pain. I've learned a lot about pain from books, but the most valuable lessons I've learned about managing pain have come from experience. I don't think any athlete can truly master pain management by other means. After all, the goal is not to avoid pain entirely. The goal is to work with pain to find your limits, and there's no one-size-fits-all blueprint for this, as each athlete's limits—which are signaled by pain—are unique and ever-changing. To succeed in using pain to guide them to their limits, athletes must figure out a lot of things for themselves by continuously listening to their bodies and monitoring their training and other factors that impact pain one way or another. It's important as well to know and understand tried-and-true training practices, as these establish a solid framework for experiential learning, but a framework is not a blueprint.

The local university in Flagstaff sometimes sends exercise physiology, physical therapy, and fitness and wellness students to my facility to serve apprenticeships. When they do, their supervisors pop in every now and again to audit my teaching. It's clear to me that they take me only half seriously, judging my practical experience far inferior to their book knowledge. The irony is that despite my lack of degrees, my knowledge of all things musculoskeletal is undebatable. Here's a fact: Our current education model delays the integration of emerging evidence into university curricula by an average of 18 years. Given this fact, self-teaching is a better—really the *only*—way to stay current in a given subject. All I care about is helping my fellow athletes and others become less limited by pain, and I believe I've developed a more effective method of caring for athletes and others through experiential knowledge coupled with current evidence-based practices. I know what I know from grinding it out in the gym and in the mountains, and while that might not get the attention of credentialed experts, it has equipped me to distinguish good, useful evidence from pseudoscience.

A LESSON IN GRIT

Every journey has its turning points, and that near-death experience at my private playground on the eastern edge of the Ouachita

Mountains became a turning point in mine. It's only a small exaggeration to say that from that day forward, I was always either climbing, training for climbing, planning a climb, or reading, talking, or at least thinking about climbing. In those days, no one really trained for climbing, but my conditioning background told me that if developing specific fitness improved performance in football and track and other sports, it ought to improve performance in climbing as well.

To that end, I built a climbing gym in my parents' hay barn. Its centerpiece was a 30-foot climbing wall that I constructed from sheets of plywood. When I learned about campus boards—a training tool invented by Wolfgang Güllich, who'd died tragically at age 31 after working as Sylvester Stallone's stunt double in the movie *Cliffhanger*—I built one of those too. Heck, I even designed my own machine for climbing-specific training, but it was too complex to fabricate on my own, so I pitched it to various manufacturers, and although there was some interest—most notably from Reebok—in the end, no one bit. I spent absurd amounts of time in that barn transforming my sprinter's body into a climber's body, my tree-trunk thighs slimming down, my hands and back getting stronger, and my weight dropping from 185 to 142 pounds.

The more I looked like a climber, the better I climbed. In bouldering, specific climbs are referred to as *problems* and range in difficulty from 0 to 17 on the V scale. Within a few months of successfully climbing my first boulder problem, I was capable of bouldering V7 (which is equivalent to 5.13 on the more familiar rope scale), having no clue how exceptional my rate of progress was until much later. In fact, my rapid progress got ahead of my body's tolerance, as I discovered the hard way one day while dangling from a 30-degree overhang with the middle digits of my right hand burrowed in a shallow two-finger pocket. Although my muscles were strong enough to complete the move, my passive tissues had some catching up to do. The flexor tendon in the proximal phalanx of my ring finger proved to be my weakest link in that moment, announcing the strain with a zap of pain that was about as intense as any I had experienced in my 24 years. I knew instantly that I had done a number on myself.

The next day, I had visible swelling in my hand and pain radiating all the way to my elbow. It hurt just to turn my hand palm up, letting the injured digit support its own weight. A week of rest brought little improvement, so I started climbing again—not as before, which was impossible, but as best I could. Through a combination of creative work-arounds and patient persistence, I advanced slowly toward full functioning, trying my best to challenge the affected tissues right up to the limit of their present tolerance and not beyond.

The process took an entire year to complete itself and included a few moments of serious self-doubt when I wondered if perhaps I ought to see someone about it. What stopped me was my still relatively fresh recollection of the fallout from my last trip to a medical professional when I was experiencing hip pain while playing high school football. In that instance, getting a diagnosis had absolutely no effect on my recovery, which my body took care of on its own, and a decidedly negative short-term effect on my anxiety level and pain-related self-efficacy. Eight years later, I knew better than to allow myself to become unnecessarily dependent on outside intervention in the same way, and today, at 49, I find myself routinely advising athletes to avoid the diagnosis trap unless they find themselves in a "red flag" scenario, which I will describe in more detail in Chapter 7.

A recent study in the journal *Skeletal Radiology* underscores the point I'm making here. A team of researchers led by Laura Horga of University College London performed MRI scans on the knees of 115 uninjured sedentary adults. Of the 230 knees scanned, 223—or 97 percent—showed abnormalities such as meniscus tears and cartilage lesions. None of the individuals involved in the study reported knee pain or dysfunction, but if one of them had, and had seen a doctor about it and gotten an MRI, they would have been diagnosed with a meniscus tear (or some other "abnormality") and prescribed treatments—perhaps even surgery—that were not only unnecessary but counterproductive. That's the diagnosis trap for you.

FALLING IS PART OF THE PROCESS

By the time my finger mishap occurred, I was no longer climbing solo, having inevitably found the handful of kindred spirits that existed in my little nook of the universe. The beginning of the end of my recreational isolation came about when a craving for steak and eggs brought me one Sunday morning to the local Waffle House, where I bumped into Jamie Anderson, a high school friend who'd awoken a similar passion for climbing during a stint in New Mexico. Naturally, the subject came up, and by the time I left the restaurant, Jamie and I had plans to meet up again and practice our newly found soulcraft together. Within a few months, Jamie and I had become the nucleus of a tight-knit posse of seven or eight zealots bonded by both climbing and our knowledge that not another soul within a 100-mile radius understood our passion.

We quickly fell into a fixed routine that held from late September until early June, when the return of Arkansas's famous sauna-like summer weather made climbing next to impossible, except at a handful of lakeside venues. Every weekend, we met up at an agreed-upon location and climbed ourselves to exhaustion, occasionally burning through enough layers of skin that small droplets of blood would suppurate to the surface of our fingertips. Then we went out drinking, my friends always putting back a few more beers than I could stomach, and parted in the wee hours having settled on our next meetup. All week long, as I baled hay or dug postholes on the farm or sold my soul at whatever big-box gym I happened to find work at, I counted the minutes till I could be back in the woods sitting beneath some stone that presented a physical challenge and a mental puzzle.

As boulderers, we were outcasts among outcasts, and we liked it that way. Most climbers prefer roped climbing, mainly because it feels safer and can allow for longer routes. Bouldering is simpler, more stripped down—just you and the rock—and that primal quality is the essence of its appeal to enthusiasts. Boulderers tend to be purists, and despite our rough-hewn ways, the guys in our little clique were deceptively principled. For example, if a particular boulder problem presented a dangerous landing or an uncomfortable hold, we took pride in either accepting the risk and discomfort or choosing to move on to something else, eschewing the compromise of modifying the site to make it safer or easier. We didn't judge ourselves better than everyone else, but we did believe we had a shared calling that held us apart from the maddening world in which we felt so out of place.

The spell we were under in those heady days derived a measure of its poignancy from our keen awareness of our situation's ephemerality. Most of us wanted to live somewhere other than where we did, so it was only a matter of time before we scattered. I wanted to get the heck out of Arkansas as much as any of us, but a part of me also didn't want the experience we were having to end. The next best thing to prolonging it, I figured, was preserving it, and to that end I bought myself a Sony Handycam and took it everywhere, recording hundreds of hours of me and the crew climbing and hanging out.

It so happened that Hot Springs hosted a major documentary film festival in October each year. And it also happened that my friend Nick had a job at a television station in nearby Conway. With minimal effort, I persuaded Nick to let me inside at night to edit the footage I'd collected into a feature-length film. When the festival rolled around, my friends and I rented out a theater and invited everyone we knew to a premier screening. I titled my debut film *The Gift*. As art, it was lacking, but as a memorial of this beautiful phase of my life, I consider it a masterpiece.

My ticket out of Hot Springs was a delivery job I took with Coca-Cola in the fall of 2000 with the specific intention of lobbying for a transfer to Flagstaff, where the company had a distribution center. I chose Flagstaff because it offered a wealth of nearby first-ascent opportunities and because I preferred its dharma-bum style to the more ego-driven, look-at-me bouldering culture that prevailed in Colorado's Front Range, where I'd made that life-changing spring break trip with my buddy John in high school. I remember lying prone on the floor of my apartment with a USGS (United States Geological Survey) topographical map spread out in front of me, scanning for concentric rings identifying a potential jewel of a climb.

The hub of Flagstaff's bouldering community was Stromboli's Pizza, where anyone who liked to climb and who wasn't a complete asshole could make friends quickly, and I darkened its doorway often in my early days in town. As a newcomer to the scene who was already able to climb with its most venerated veterans, I found myself in an odd place in the pecking order. It was a bit like moving to town as an unknown 2:14 marathoner. Such a person would almost *have to* train with the few runners in town of equal ability, yet he'd still have to earn their respect one workout at a time.

In the movie of my life, there will be a scene where I take on a Flagstaff boulderer's rite of passage: a so-called roof problem known as the Receptionist. The reason boulderers refer to climbs as *problems* is that you must solve them to complete them. Strength and skill alone won't suffice. You have to figure out where to put your hands and feet and which specific techniques to use at each step from the bottom to the top. That's why boulderers are big on first ascents—climbing problems no one has solved yet—and on advancing up the V scale of difficulty. To boulder is to spend more time falling than climbing. It is a sport for the patient. Boulderers have been known to spend years trying to master a single move that's standing in the way of their solving a particular problem.

A roof problem is one that features a horizontal section. The Receptionist is categorized as a V10, a grade that was climbed far less often 20-plus years ago than it is today, but it was well within my ability. My goal was to on-sight the problem, or complete it on my first attempt, which is a way of trying to match the thrill you get from a first ascent on a problem that's merely new to you. I failed on the very last move, which was better than all but a few climbers had done in their first crack at the Receptionist and thus earned me a measure of respect and local clout. I had reached a level of bouldering that allowed me to climb many classic problems around the country and abroad, following in the footsteps of my climbing heroes and occasionally climbing with those heroes—the likes of Fredrick Nicole and Chris Sharma—some of whom I remain good friends with.

Having read John Sherman's bible of bouldering, I had a sense of how eccentric the key personalities were and how off-center the culture produced by the interaction of these quirky individuals was. Things have changed quite a bit in the past couple of decades, but back then, climbing in general and the bouldering community in particular were peopled by zealots who loved the sport so much they were willing to make almost any sacrifice to do it as much as possible—a.k.a. dirtbags. A good example of the type was my friend Tim Doyle, a Canadian who figured out how to survive on $2 a day and did so for years on end. In fact, as far as I know, he's still doing it, though inflation may have increased his per diem to 4 bucks.

Others tried to get by on even less. I met some German boulderers who wanted to pass a climbing season in the United States and came to the conclusion that the only way they could make it work was to live on monkey food—as in the stuff that laboratory monkeys are fed. I have no idea how they came up with this notion, much less how they got their hands on a four-month supply of monkey food. What I do know is that they got so impacted by the stuff that they had to call off the experiment and beat a hasty retreat back to the fatherland.

PERSISTENCE AND PATIENCE

When I look back on those times from my current vantage, I'm struck that although pain of some form was a constant companion for my climbing friends, and although bona fide injuries were not uncommon, few of them ever saw a doctor about anything nontraumatic in nature. The primary reason, no doubt, was that they couldn't afford to. Health insurance was almost as rare as teetotaling in our tribe. In retrospect, I see this privation as an advantage because it all but forced climbers to be self-reliant in managing pain and injuries, and most learned to do so with a great deal of success. Each learned to balance persistence and patience, using pain as a guide toward their present limits, taking every inch their body would give them and not an inch more.

There were exceptions, of course. One time, my friend Chris Lee hurt his elbow playing ultimate frisbee and quickly discovered that the issue affected his climbing. Rightly considered one of the smartest and wisest members of our group, Chris had a master's in chemistry and wrote SAT questions for a living. Science clearly supports remaining active during injury, which is proven to reduce pain, accelerate healing, maintain function, promote self-efficacy, and even reduce inflammation. But most medical professionals recommend rest, and Chris did what was recommended, spending the majority of our climbing season on the sidelines. Predictably, he got nothing for it. Recognizing he was making a mistake, I urged Chris to dust off his climbing shoes and start climbing again, and when he did, he quickly got better. I don't mean to throw my friend under the bus. Chris would tell you himself that an excess of caution only prolonged his recovery.

A different sort of exception was John Sherman, the aforementioned bouldering pioneer and V scale inventor. I finally met John in 2003 at Kelly Canyon, a treasure trove of undiscovered sandstone cliffs and boulders that my friends and I had spent the last couple years exploring and scouting for future adventures. I was working on a problem called the Incredible Undercling when a guy bearing a strong resemblance to John walked up and began to observe. The next time I fell, I did what any fan would do.

"Are you John Sherman?" I asked.

"I used to be," he answered.

At the time, John was 44 years old, yet he moved like a much older man—and one who hadn't taken very good care of himself. In concession to chronic low-back pain, he stood and walked with a dowager's stoop. It was shocking to see. This icon of the sport literally couldn't even stand up straight! In a sense, he really hadn't taken very good care of himself—not in the usual sense of being inactive and eating too much processed food but by placing a lot of stress on his body through his bouldering exploits without properly managing that stress through supplemental training and musculoskeletal care. Worse, in his search for solutions and explanations for his pain and loss of function, John had put himself in the hands of doctors and therapists who had taught him to believe that his shoulders and back suffered from "degenerative changes," which is the medicalized name for wear and tear.

The thing about wear and tear is that it doesn't actually exist. At least not in the sense that many believe it does. The truth is that throughout life, the human body retains the capacity to repair the wear it experiences. Athletes find themselves in the state in which John found himself at age 44 not because they have overused certain tissues and thereby broken them down in irreversible ways but because those natural repair processes have been stymied by mistakes, including an all-or-nothing approach to continued activity. Little did I know when I shook John's hand that day in 2003 that I was just a few months away from developing the shoulder pain that would result in my own misguided indoctrination in the structural model of pain. For that very reason, oddly, I was in a better position then to help John Sherman become John Sherman again than I would have been a year or two later. But I didn't make the offer, for although I was no longer the greenhorn from Arkansas fresh off the turnip truck, I had no credentials to back up my experience-based knowledge, and John was a superstar of the sport who didn't know me from Adam.

With other climbers, I was less reticent. Within the rarefied club of elite boulderers, I developed a reputation as the guy who trained on nonclimbing days, which is now common but back then was the kind of thing that provoked teasing. Wherever we went to set up camp and climb for a season—whether it was Yosemite, Switzerland, El Paso, or closer to home—I found a climbing wall and whatever else I needed to stay on top of my conditioning. Such behavior could not possibly have passed unnoticed, and a few among those who did notice—and who perhaps connected the behavior to my continuing improvement as a boulderer—began to tag along so that in time, I was surrounded by a small crew of fellow training dorks. Most of them, I believe, would say they got the same benefits I got from the commitment we made. My friend Clint Hill, for example, saw the stress tolerance of his shoulders increase markedly during his time as my workout buddy.

Coaching my fellow athletes remained a side hustle for me, however, until 2010, when circumstances left me with little choice but to go all in. When the Great Recession hit, I lost my job as a health teacher, a financial blow that was perfectly timed for maximum negative impact. Betsy had just left the work field to go back to school for interior design, and we had just bought a home together, so when Betsy's student loan funds arrived, we used them to rent a warehouse and open Paragon Athletics. Like any new business that's launched on shoestring capital with zero advance planning, ours struggled initially. But the faithful few early clients who gave us a chance got good enough results from my nascent Training as Treatment approach that the resulting word-of-mouth referrals allowed us to survive and eventually grow.

RESTORING A LEGEND

When John Sherman walked into the facility a year later wearing a baggy tracksuit and beat-up Velcro track shoes, smelling of malt liquor and weighing a good 40 pounds more than he had when I first met him, Paragon Athletics was thriving. In fact, John interrupted a group workout with more than two dozen attendees—or would have done so if I hadn't made him wait.

His appearance wasn't wholly unexpected. Two years earlier, I had finally mustered the gumption to offer to help John get his mojo back. The moment he entered Paragon, I knew he was ready to take me up on the offer and that he was ready because he was desperate. Recently diagnosed with a torn labrum in his left shoulder, John was scheduled for surgery, but having lost much of his prior faith in doctors, he wanted to give my way a try before he went under the knife. A lot had changed since our initial encounter, however. John was now 56 years old and in even rougher shape than before. I had found my true vocational mission and was singularly devoted to it. Helping John certainly fit into this mission, but he was a special case—an all-time great climber with sky-high ambitions who needed and deserved intensive support. With someone like him, you have to be in for a pound if you're in for a penny. I told him I'd think about it.

In the end, I couldn't resist, and John and I started working together two weeks later. My first priority was to give him a much-needed reality check. John still thought of himself as one of the most capable boulderers on the planet, and although I truly believed he could be great again, I saw more clearly than he did just how far he had to go. So I handed him a jump rope and asked him to show me how many jumps he could complete without interruption. That number turned out to be zero.

"John, you are a threadbare man," I said to him.

Harsh, I know, but there was a method to the madness. As a coach, you have to handle each athlete individually, tailoring your messaging to meet their specific needs. In John's case, the need was for full buy-in to the slow stepwise process I had in mind for him. Having made my point, I told him to give me nine months to work my magic, which sounded like an eternity to John but seemed terrifyingly optimistic to me—a timeline achievable only if everything went perfectly, and maybe not even then.

We'd only been at it for a few weeks when John made a trip to Yosemite to test himself against Midnight Lightning, a V8 considered the world's most famous bouldering problem. He couldn't even get off the ground, unable to complete the first of 50 required moves. It was a stinging humiliation—far more humbling than the rope-jumping fail—but it served as another reality check that pushed John to accept a more patient approach to his comeback.

In that first phase of the project, the stuff I had John do didn't look much like exercise. I was focused on desensitization, more or less tricking his brain into expecting less pain when he used his shoulder. I might have him lie down, for example, and move his arm in an overhead pressing motion, confirm that he felt no pain, and then inform him that he had just used his shoulder in the same way that invariably caused pain when he did it standing upright. Over time, such expectancy violations created new associative links that enabled John to do more and more without discomfort.

Meanwhile, I brought John along with equal care with respect to his understanding of and belief in my Training as Treatment approach and its theoretical foundation, the biopsychosocial pain model. When the moment seemed right, I dropped little breadcrumbs of research, trusting that his innate skepticism would compel him to secretly fact-check me, inevitably affirming the veracity of what I'd told him.

Nine months—almost to the day—after our first session together, John returned to Midnight Lightning and made it all the way to the final move of the problem, stunning the bouldering world. Now 61 years old, John is even stronger than he was that day—as strong as he's ever been, he claims. Yet he still hasn't conquered Midnight Lighting—not because he can't but because there are so few opportunities (perfect conditions are needed, and they don't happen often) and because, as I mentioned earlier, to boulder is to spend more time falling than climbing. John broke his ankle one year, tore an Achilles tendon another year, injured a finger another year, and suffered a full-thickness tear to the subscapularis tendon of his left shoulder another year—bad-luck injuries that proper conditioning can only do so much to prevent.

Incidentally, after John's shoulder tendon was surgically repaired, I asked the surgeon how the labrum looked, having talked John into canceling the surgery he was scheduled to have for that issue when we started working together.

"The labrum?" he asked. "It looked beautiful. Not a thing wrong with it."

THE THEATER OF PAIN

In the summer of 2004, more than nine months into my struggle with shoulder pain, I made an appointment to see Dr. Hope (a pseudonym), a physical therapist in Flagstaff that I found neither by his reputation nor via personal referral but through the phone book—I was that desperate. The consultation began with a familiar question asked by clinicians who see people with athletic pain and injury: "So what brings you in today?"

"I'm here," I announced, "to interview another therapist."

To his credit, Dr. Hope laughed. But I wasn't joking. Having already seen five other physical therapists and chiropractors about the same problem, none of whom had been able to help me, I was beginning to lose faith in these professions. In fact, if anything, the folks I'd sought help from thus far had actually made matters worse. A couple of them had at least told me what they thought was wrong with my body—that my trapezius muscles were overactive, for example, or that I had displaced ribs—but this information served only to exacerbate my feeling of powerlessness in relation to the problem. One particular chiropractor had warned me not to move my shoulder for 24 hours after he performed an adjustment, an unnecessary caution that merely amplified my fear of using the joint. No one, however, had been able to shed any light on why the shoulder hurt or make it hurt any less, and I was getting frustrated.

Dr. Hope took me through the usual intake process and evaluation, then recommended a combination of soft tissue work and traction. The soft tissue treatment amounted to little more than a glorified shoulder rub but was just different enough from a Swedish massage in technique and pleasantness that I assumed Dr. Hope knew what he was doing. The traction inspired confidence in a different way. I was strapped into a kooky little machine that grabbed me by the neck and tried to separate my head from my body—or so it felt. I figured that some serious thought must have gone into the design and construction of such a weird contraption.

Like his predecessors, Dr. Hope did not offer a definitive diagnosis, but when I researched the treatments he'd chosen for me, I deduced that he must have suspected a case of thoracic outlet syndrome, a condition involving compressed nerves or blood vessels. Knowing what I know today, I do not believe I had thoracic outlet syndrome at the time, nor do I believe that soft tissue manipulations and traction machines are reliable treatments for any condition, but I cannot deny that my shoulder pain did begin to abate during the three weeks I spent in the care of Dr. Hope.

Pain is such a complex phenomenon that there's really no telling why the beginning of the end of this frustrating episode came when it did. If I had to guess, I would say that a decline in allostatic load had something to do with it. I've mentioned already that life stress likely made a significant contribution to the onset of pain during the winter I spent in Arkansas after the Butter Bean breakdown incident in Winfield, Alabama. My subsequent return to Flagstaff had lifted a weight off my shoulders, so to speak, and I was also feeling content in my new job as a manager at a coffee shop that had supplanted Stromboli's as the main hangout for climbers. Betsy and I were also enjoying our new accommodations: a cozy little town house that was a significant upgrade from the ramshackle cabin we'd shared in Hot Springs, where we slept on a sheet of plywood.

In the context of these welcome changes, it's possible that just about any clinician I might have chosen to see at that time would have turned out to be the one in whose care I started on the road to recovery. Dr. Hope deserves credit for instilling in me some confidence in the treatments he administered. They may have been pure theater, but they were convincing theater for me at that moment and perhaps effective for this reason.

Overall, though, my encounters with the sports medicine establishment continued to leave a bad taste in my mouth. Sure, my shoulder had gotten better eventually, but the process had taken almost an entire year, and that year had been filled with frustration. I hated the thought of other athletes having to go through similar experiences, and I made a silent vow to do what I could to spare as many of them as I could. In fact, I fixed my mind on preventing virtually *all* nontraumatic athletic injuries, and I was convinced it was possible. Sports performance was and is still my passion, but injury prevention became my obsession in the wake of my personal experience with prolonged dysfunction.

My conviction that I could succeed in this mission rested on two supporting beliefs, one of which I still hold today, the other of which I am frankly embarrassed to have ever held. I remain convinced that athletes do not belong in orthopedic offices and physical therapy clinics unless they've suffered a traumatic injury of some kind (e.g., a bone fracture). They belong instead in the gym with a knowledgeable coach like me. With proper training, athletes simply don't need help from doctors or physical therapists unless they find themselves in a red-flag scenario. Where I went wrong was in accepting the sports medicine establishment's own structural model of injury as the basis for the gym-based musculoskeletal care I offered to athletes early on.

MY REGRETTABLE DETOUR INTO
THE STRUCTURAL MODEL

As you've learned, the structural model asserts that athletic injuries are caused by incorrect movements that, in turn, are caused by imbalances in the musculoskeletal system or by exceeding tissue tolerance. Given that all the experts I knew subscribed to this model, I bought into it as well, not recognizing that the whole thing was a house of cards lacking scientific legitimacy. So I asked myself, If athletic injuries are indeed caused by incorrect movements that, in turn, are caused by imbalances in the musculoskeletal system, what's stopping me and other trainers from preventing injuries from ever happening by correcting incorrect movements and balancing the musculoskeletal systems of athletes?

The only obstacle standing in my way at that moment—or so I believed—was lack of knowledge, so I embarked on a furious quest to learn everything there was to know about nontraumatic athletic injuries, the scores of different diagnostics used to identify them, biomechanics, functional anatomy, and eventually pain, on the assumption that pain equals injury. Ironically, it was this very quest for knowledge that ultimately awakened me to the fact that the current methods of treating pain and injury were a whole lot of smoke and mirrors, but it didn't happen right away. On the contrary, for too long I looked past obvious signs that the structural story didn't stand up to scrutiny and became a willing actor in the theater that perpetuated it.

As an outsider to the sports medicine establishment, I did not have an easy time learning everything there was to know about keeping athletes healthy. Today's bounty of online resources—such as ResearchGate, an online community made up of forward-thinking academics—allows autodidacts like me to access all the important scientific journals with the click of a button. But in the dark ages of 2005 to 2013, I had to schlep around to bone up on my areas of interest, going from the Northern Arizona University (NAU) library, where I probably spent more time than 99 percent of enrolled students, to professional conferences all over the map, where, with my high school education and my personal trainer certificate, I stood out like a linebacker at a ballet lesson, but I didn't care. In Reston, Virginia, I absorbed the latest discoveries about human connective tissue at the annual Fascia Research Congress. Later that year, in Carpentaria, California, I participated in a workshop led by Robert Schleip, who was visiting the United States from the University of Ulm in Germany to share his world-leading knowledge about joint structure and function. Can you guess how many other supergeeks besides myself attended both of these events? That's right: zero.

Somewhere along the way, I became infatuated with running biomechanics. This was probably inevitable given the abundance of runners in Flagstaff, the famously high rate of injury in the sport, and the plenteous research being done on the causes and prevention of running-related injuries. I purchased, read, reread, and in the end virtually memorized a book that bore the definitive title *Human Locomotion*: a 400-plus page colossus featuring more than 500 anatomical drawings. Written by a chiropractor who specialized in the prevention and treatment of running injuries, the book is a triumph of structural thinking. Chapter 3, titled "Ideal Motions During the Gait Cycle," presents a breathtakingly detailed set of standards for how the body *should* look when running. The glaring fact that few, if any, flesh-and-blood humans actually run in this supposedly ideal manner did not seem to trouble the authors. In their view, it was the clinician's job to point out the flaws in each individual runner's technique and structure and, if possible, make the necessary corrections for optimal movement. I fully bought into this way of thinking, and I was soon telling the runners I worked with what was wrong with their movements and muscles.

But wait, there's more. My plunge down the rabbit hole of running biomechanics led me to gait clinics where more was said about the human running stride than any runner would think possible. I then discovered a pair of running-form gurus who presented similar material online in the form of high-quality videos and well-crafted articles. Blinded by confirmation bias—the natural human tendency to focus on evidence that seems to support what we already believe and to ignore evidence that challenges our beliefs—I absorbed this material with the same lack of skepticism. To my everlasting regret, it wasn't only the substance but also the style of these two icons of structural thinking that I passed on to my athletes during this period. Their steady stream of slick content created an aura of omniscience concerning what a runner's feet and legs and other body parts should look like, how much range of motion their joints should have, how strong their joints should be, how they should move, and of course, what they should look like when they run, down to the most minute detail. A subtle tone of condescension pervaded every sentence of these stride gurus, amplifying an air of authority, at least for the susceptible.

The people who know me best would affirm that I am neither arrogant nor condescending by nature, but I took care to emulate the gurus' structure-and-function shtick at the gym during this phase. If you had come to me then with plantar fasciitis or a sore Achilles tendon or some other common runner's complaint, you would have been subjected to a very different experience than you'd get if you came to me with the same issues today. From the moment you walked in the door, I would have tried to demonstrate everything I knew about biomechanics. Specifically, I would have asked you to remove the insoles from your shoes and then studied them like tea leaves, amazing you (or not) with all the clues I saw in them. I might even have inspected your toenails and explained to you what their formation told me about your running form.

For my next trick, I would have ordered you to perform various actions—stand up, lie down, squat as deeply as you can—scrutinizing your movement and telling you many things you never knew about various parts of your anatomy. There's a test called Craig's Test, for example, where you lie prone on a treatment table with your knees bent to 90 degrees and the clinician manually rotates your leg outward. I would have been sure to let you know if your angle of femoral anteversion failed to fall within the normal range of 8 to 15 degrees. These diagnostic tests can actually be useful as retest tools to see how someone's pain is changing, but that's not how I was using them. At that time, I was oblivious to the fact that Craig's Test is completely lacking in diagnostic or predictive validity.

Unfortunately, this was the equivalent of working with fat calipers all over again. Except this time, I didn't recognize what I was doing. When I used fat calipers on a client as a rookie personal trainer, I understood that they served no purpose other than to objectify the person they were applied to. I had sworn then never to repeat that mistake, yet here I was years later, once again administering unsubstantiated tools and methods that accomplished nothing more than to foster a completely unhelpful relationship between me and the people I was trying to help.

I remember one client in particular. Her only mistake was walking into the gym on a day when, for whatever reason, I was feeling especially superior and dogmatic. A runner, she seemed nervous and perhaps somewhat intimidated from the outset, and I did all the right things to make her feel even more so. Instead of engaging her in a relaxed, caring conversation about her running and her life, her concerns and her hopes, I threw her straight into the usual tests, told her what a disaster her squat performance was, and described the long and daunting process she would have to undergo in order for me to fix her. It's no surprise that she never returned, and when eventually I came to my senses, I vowed to apologize if I ever saw her again.

The term *overcoaching*, which Merriam-Webster defines as "coach[ing] (someone) to an excessive degree," describes me to a T circa 2007. With the best of intentions, believing that I was saving athletes from accidental self-harm, I drew attention to every little flaw I could detect in the way they executed everything from squats to climbs. They didn't even have to be my clients to receive my sage advice.

There was a climbing gym located next door to Paragon Athletics. One time, I popped in there and noticed a young woman I knew just well enough to say hello. She was doing a particular abdominal exercise with excessive lumbar spine extension. Unsolicited, I pointed out her error, warning her that over time, it could lead to back issues. The woman sort of blew me off, and she was right to do so, for it is now a firmly established fact that what she was doing is not at all harmful.

DIFFERENT BODIES MOVE DIFFERENTLY

Had I been born a few years later than I was, I might never have taken this regrettable detour into structuralism. Although science never supported its core tenets, there's a difference between lack of evidence and contradictory evidence, and the last decade or so has brought an avalanche of powerful evidence directly contradicting the notion that there is only one right way to move and all other ways lead to injury.

Let's go back to running injuries, the things that lured me down the structuralist rabbit hole in the first place with their sheer commonness and my earnest desire to make them less common. In 2020, the *Scandinavian Journal of Medicine and Science in Sports* published the results of a study by Finnish and Canadian researchers that used machine learning to analyze the stride patterns of 291 runners and attempted to correlate specific patterns to certain types of injury as well as to overall injury risk. They found no such correlations, an unexpected result that led the authors to speculate that "there is not a single 'protective gait pattern' reducing the likelihood of developing running-related injuries." In other words, there is no single correct way to run to avoid injury. Nor, for that matter, is there a single right way to perform any other athletic movement. Each person's body is unique, and although there is a place for technique instruction in sports training, there is a much bigger place for learning by doing, a process that overcoaching actively thwarts.

Returning to the example of the woman I observed performing an abdominal exercise with excessive lumbar spine extension, I'd like to point out that she was, in fact, doing the movement suboptimally from a pure efficacy perspective. If I had a client who did the same thing today, I would suggest she consider adjusting her technique to enhance the benefit of the exercise, but I would present this information carefully. In these situations, it's important to avoid creating fear around the movement—or worse, provoking a nocebo (pain-suggesting) effect. This is a well-established phenomenon that has more evidence for causing pain than biomechanics. And if I saw a nonclient doing the same suboptimal movement, I would keep my mouth shut and mind my own business, realizing that although they may be missing some performance gain, the athlete isn't hurting themself.

All of this came later, however. In the structuralist phase of my career, it wasn't enough for me to save every athlete I encountered in person from injuries that were supposedly caused by ostensibly incorrect movement patterns. I wanted to save every athlete in the world. To that end, I began to write a book that would deliver my approach to the masses. The idea was to offer a comprehensive set of self-administered tests that readers could use to determine whether they had a normal, healthy range of motion and adequate strength throughout their bodies. I collected and organized exercises to correct every problem an athlete might encounter. I believed—or convinced myself, anyway—that if I did my job, any athlete who committed to my approach would be all but immune to nontraumatic musculo-skeletal pain and injury.

The book was published in May 2013 and exceeded my wildest hopes, at least commercially. It became a *New York Times* bestseller, was translated into several different languages, and went through three editions. The catch is that I didn't write it—Kelly Starrett did. That's right: I was scooped! Normally, getting beat to the printer is a would-be author's worst nightmare, but in this particular case, I wasn't even remotely disappointed that Kelly—a German-born, California-based physical therapist and CrossFit trainer—got my message out ahead of me because by then, it was no longer my message. The house of cards was beginning to fall.

UNCOVERING CONFIRMATION BIAS

I wish I could say it was personal experience that caused me to realize that the structural model of pain and injury was wrong. After all, the ultimate proof of its falseness is the fact that forcing athletes to conform to theoretically ideal movement patterns does *not* reduce injury risk, and there I was at the gym, forcing athletes to move the way structuralist doctrine said everyone should move, and they were still getting injured.

Except they weren't—not most of them, anyway. If the biopsychosocial model I now endorse has taught us anything, it's that pain responds to myriad influences and that no influence has a more ameliorative effect on pain than exercise. For these reasons—coupled with my all-too-human bias toward confirming what I already believed—it was difficult for me to see the cracks in the foundation of structuralism. Without knowing it, I was doing a lot of things right: keeping my clients active despite their pain, believing in their ability to overcome their pain and communicating that belief, caring about their well-being and expressing it. Although my methods were far from perfect, they were good enough to achieve positive results in the majority of my clients despite the negative impact of structuralism. This is why, like any other individual practitioner, I needed the help of something bigger than personal experience—namely, science—to see the truth.

In essence, science is little more than a formalized good-faith effort to overcome our natural tendency to believe what we want to believe. Its methods don't guarantee we're always right, but they do guarantee we're never wrong forever. The flip side of this reality, of course, is that what science suggests is true at any given time is likely to change in the future. To embrace science, then, is to accept that you're probably going to have to change your mind at some point in the future.

Unfortunately, many scientific errors persist longer than they should, including the great and consequential error of structuralism. That's because not all science is good science. For example, in 1944, the physician and biomechanist Verne Inman published the results of a study involving a single subject that was somehow allowed to become the basis for diagnosing a condition known as scapular dyskinesis. Measurements taken on just one person were used to establish a universal standard for *scapulohumeral rhythm*, or motion at the shoulder joint. This never should have happened, yet to this day, most physical therapists are taught that the scapula and humerus need to move in a precise ratio or else pain and injury (i.e., scapular dyskinesis) are likely. Given its dubious origin, it's unsurprising that this diagnosis maps poorly to shoulder pain and dysfunction. Lots of people whose shoulders fit the accepted definition of scapular dyskinesis are asymptomatic, and lots of people who have scapular dyskinesis and shoulder pain are able to overcome the pain without any change to the condition that supposedly caused it.

Mind you, this is just one example of structuralism's flimsy foundation—there are literally dozens of other equally questionable physical examinations that clinicians routinely use to diagnose pathologies in the shoulder joint alone. In a comprehensive review of past studies assessing the reliability of these tests that was published in the journal *Physiotherapy* in 2010, researchers at Sheffield Hallam University concluded with brutal succinctness that "there is no consistent evidence that any examination procedure used in shoulder assessments has acceptable levels of reliability." And subsequent research into the validity of such diagnostics has only raised more doubt.

What's going on here? How is it possible that a global paradigm of standard practice for diagnosing and treating nontraumatic musculoskeletal injuries could exist with very little valid scientific backing? To answer this question would require me to go deeper into the philosophy of science than you probably want me to. What I will say is that it's not some greed-fueled conspiracy to part athletic rubes from their money. The vast majority of clinicians who are perpetuating the structural paradigm are themselves victims of the hoax, as I myself once was. Indeed, it's not really a hoax but an honest mistake that exploits certain vulnerabilities affecting every field of science.

Consider, for example, the idea that exercise-related muscle cramps are caused by dehydration. This idea goes back to 1932, when John Talbott, a physician with the Fatigue Laboratory at Harvard University, traveled to Nevada in the hope of figuring out why so many of the workers involved in building the Hoover Dam were suffering from muscle cramps. Talbott observed that cramping workers had lost high levels of body fluid and electrolyte minerals through sweat. He noted also that the cramps seemed to abate when the workers were given salted milk to drink. On the basis of these observations, Talbott deduced that muscle cramps were caused by dehydration and electrolyte depletion, a conclusion he shared in a highly influential paper published in the *Journal of Clinical Investigation*. Talbott was a respected scientist, after all, and the explanation he proposed seemed plausible and bore an elegant simplicity.

Decades later, when the running boom hit and suddenly marathoners were cramping up left and right, the theory that dehydration causes muscle cramps became official doctrine in organizations such as the American College of Sports Medicine, which issued hydration and electrolyte intake guidelines for athletes, coaches, trainers, and others. This codification of the theory gave it a stickiness that was amplified by sports drink brands whose products were designed to prevent and treat dehydration and its supposed consequences.

The problem was that the original study upon which this paradigm was built lacked a control group, a cardinal scientific error that stripped Talbott's findings of any validity. Only when skeptical researchers went back to the study, noticed this flaw, and then conducted their own properly controlled experiments was it discovered that dehydration is not, in fact, a significant cause of muscle cramps during exercise.

You'd be amazed how often this sort of thing happens, and again, the reason it happens so often is that not all science is good science. The first key vulnerability of any scientific discipline is that new findings don't appear in a vacuum. Instead, they appear within a social context shaped by existing belief paradigms, intellectual trends, and other factors that cause scientists to be less skeptical of some ideas than they are of others, just as the physiologists of John Talbott's day were relatively uncritical of the notion that dehydration caused muscle cramps. As the philosopher of science Karl Popper put it, "Thinking people tend to develop some framework into which they try to fit whatever new idea they may come across; as a rule, they even translate any new idea which they meet into a language appropriate to their own framework. One of the most characteristic tasks of philosophy is to attack, if necessary, the framework itself."

This is easier said than done, however, because another key vulnerability of science is that just like the rest of us, scientists don't like admitting they were wrong or changing their minds. Thus, when a new idea becomes an old idea, scientists (and scientific organizations like the American College of Sports Medicine) become protective of it, warding off attacks from newer ideas that challenge it. This conservative propensity in science becomes exacerbated by a third vulnerability: a tendency for material interests to develop around established belief paradigms. When a new idea literally threatens people's jobs and companies' bottom lines (think Gatorade in the case of the dehydration theory of muscle cramping), those who stand to lose something stop caring whether the new idea is true or not.

DECONSTRUCTING THE STRUCTURAL MODEL

The structural model of injury has followed the same pattern as the dehydration theory of cramping. When it took root in the middle of the 20th century, the way had been prepared for it by the triumph of a mechanistic view of human anatomy that had come to the fore more than a century earlier. In much the same manner that the computer age would later lead neuroscientists and psychologists to draw fraught parallels between brains and computers, physiologists of the machine age couldn't resist the temptation to apply a machine model to human anatomy and function. This conceptual framework rendered them less skeptical than they ought to have been of the proposition that nontraumatic sports injuries are caused by flawed movement patterns rooted in structural imbalances. Consequently, faulty research like the previously mentioned study on scapular dyskinesis was given a pass, and in due time, the structural model was being taught in orthopedic and physical therapy classrooms all over the world. Indeed, the discipline of physical therapy as we know it is predicated on this model.

Athletes are not merely innocent witnesses in the theater of sports medicine and physical therapy as it's currently practiced—they play an active role. When athletes who are experiencing pain put themselves in the hands of a clinician, they expect a certain kind of show. Specifically, they want the diagnostic and treatment processes to *feel* scientific. Medical jargon, high-tech instruments, and seemingly precise measurements inspire confidence in the care they are receiving, as they did for me in Dr. Hope's office.

Clinicians aren't knowingly deceiving athletes when, for example, they use a micrometer to take anatomical measurements—a practice that serves no useful purpose whatsoever. As I mentioned in Chapter 2, scientists and doctors themselves are biased toward things that bear the trappings of science whether or not these things are actually scientific. Nor is this bias limited to the medical sphere. In the wake of the 9/11 terrorist attacks in the United States, transportation safety experts studied various ways of improving the security of air travel. One of the things they discovered was that simply talking to passengers was more effective in identifying malefactors than high-tech scanners were, but both the government and industry groups went with scanners because they made passengers feel safer than low-tech human-to-human interaction did. Similarly, we are all to blame, to some degree, for perpetuating the structural model of athletic injury even in light of growing evidence against it.

Again, though, what makes science special is not that it's never wrong but that it's self-correcting. The incentive structures that function to preserve ill-founded beliefs are counterbalanced by incentive structures that lead to the inevitable exposure of the falsity of such beliefs. Sooner or later, there's bound to come along a researcher with no particular attachment to an existing belief and with much to gain from being credited as the person who put forward a truer truth. In the case of the structural model of athletic injury, it was a revolution in pain science that brought the whole house of cards toppling down.

THE ROLE OF PAIN IN PERFORMANCE

Earlier in my career, I viewed injuries as problems to be fixed and regarded pain as a mere epiphenomenon—nothing more than a symptom of an injury's existence and an indicator of its severity. But in fact, pain is a phenomenon unto itself, and as such, it merits treatment as a discreet object of study. In the 1970s, scientists who studied pain began to realize that the relationship between pain and injury was a lot looser than was previously believed, a realization that led to the development of the biopsychosocial model of pain. At the same time, skeptics of the structural model of injury kept poking holes in the flimsy research supporting it. Together, these two factors removed the blindfold from the eyes of clinicians like me. If we truly wanted to keep athletes healthy, we would need to be open to whichever methods appeared to work best.

I discovered the biopsychosocial model of pain through Greg Lehman in 2013. By then, I had begun to see that the emperor had no clothes. The specific event that brought me to Greg was a hunt for information on technique for the deep squat exercise, part of a larger effort to compile standards from musculoskeletal diagnostic tests so that I could use them preemptively, to avoid injury (pain). But while doing so, I came to the realization that the tests were rather dodgy. Indeed, it's estimated that somewhere between 93 and 96 percent of them lack clinical utility. Nevertheless, I was still doggedly searching for tests that actually worked when I came across Greg's website, where a whole new world of ideas was opened up to me. Greg is a Canadian physiotherapist, chiropractor, and strength and conditioning specialist (and occasional foreword writer, I should add) who, in addition to working one-on-one with athletes and other clients, does a lot of blogging, some research, and a good bit of travel and public speaking. He knows plenty about biomechanics—and yes, I did find some good information about the deep squat on his website—but he also has a keen interest in pain, and he was way ahead of me in embracing the biopsychosocial model and applying it in his clinical work.

At the time I found Greg, he had recently posted an article titled "Your Cranky Nerves: A Primer for Patients to Understand Pain." Under the subhead "Damage Does Not Always Equal Pain," Greg wrote the following:

> The idea that lots of pain equals lots of damage is a very difficult concept to shake. It is entrenched in how we think about pain, arthritis, surgery and injuries. When we have pain we want to know what is causing it. We assume there must be something damaged . . . that causes our pain. The problem with this is that the majority of us are walking around with some degenerative joint disease, disc protrusions, tears in our shoulder rotator cuff and all kinds of things that look like damage yet we have no pain. Conversely, you can have a lot of pain and all the imaging shows that there is no damage.

As I would soon come to appreciate, Greg was quite right in asserting that these ideas are very difficult for many people—not just athletes but clinicians and scientists as well—to assimilate. But I was ready for them. The biopsychosocial model of pain resonated with my lived experience, making theoretical sense of everything from the inability of several clinicians to find any true injury underlying my shoulder pain to the ability of many elite boulderers to stay relatively healthy and manage pain without the help of doctors or physical therapists.

I won't deny that it stung a little to realize how wrong I had been to accept the structural model of athletic injury so uncritically, but this feeling was more than made up for by my excitement about the science of pain. It was kind of like getting out of a bad relationship that I didn't quite realize was bad until my true soulmate came along. Pain science opened up a treasure trove of learning opportunities for me.

My overall approach to learning didn't change. As before, it entailed following conceptual breadcrumbs that were dropped in Facebook discussion groups, in YouTube videos, by the doctors I interacted with in my work with athletes, and elsewhere. A physician might say something about the inflammatory process, for example, and I would take the opportunity to learn everything there was to know about it. But in the course of reading up on inflammation, I might come across repeated references to, say, confidence intervals—another breadcrumb, this one leading me to bone up on statistics.

None of this learning was done for its own sake, of course. My goal was to apply it in the gym in the service of my mission to help athletes stay healthy and perform better. It wasn't long before I began to see concrete proof that the practical application of the biopsychosocial model of pain to athlete training was game-changing. Among the earliest beneficiaries of my new learning was Jenn, a serious climber with chronic low-back pain who, though not yet 30 years old at the time, had been told by doctors that she suffered from advanced arthritis. She'd been sleeping on a heating pad every night for eight years.

Within a few months of our beginning to work together, Jenn had ditched the heating pad and was climbing as well as she ever had. Although we did plenty of strength work, that piece of my new approach to coaching was nothing new for her, except in certain details. What *was* new was the alternative way of understanding her pain experience that I spooned into Jenn's brain a drop at a time, and it made all the difference. Jenn is exactly the sort of athlete I was likely to have failed to help when I remained mired in structuralism and whose lack of progress I would have blamed not on structuralism but on my own lack of complete mastery of the model and its applications. But I did not fail with Jenn. Her back still gives her some trouble every now and again, but when it does, she works through it using the methods that I now collectively refer to as Training as Treatment.

5

TRAINING AS TREATMENT

A few years ago, I started using the hashtag #trainingastreatment in some of my social media posts. I'm not big on marketing and branding, but I needed a name for my approach to pain management, and what I came up with does a pretty good job of encapsulating my mission to replace medical treatment with physical training as the dominant method for managing athletic pain.

My previous approach to helping athletes could have been called training *and* treatment. Even in the days when I bought into the structural model of injury, I believed that gym work had a significant role to play in athletic pain management. But back then, I saw that role as being distinct from and, in a sense, subordinate to that of medical treatment. It was this way of thinking that led me to decide to collaborate with a physical therapist to work alongside me when Paragon Athletics relocated in 2012. My vision was to make the facility a kind of one-stop shop for musculoskeletal care for athletes. And that's precisely what it is today—only without a physical therapist on staff. My vision hasn't changed, you see. What *did* change was my belief that training and treatment are separate processes, each requiring its own special expertise.

The main driver of this evolution was my immersion in pain science. The more I read, the better I understood which methods of athletic pain management were supported by solid evidence and which were not. And the better I understood what does and doesn't work to manage athletic pain, the less need I saw for a physical therapy partner to fulfill Paragon's mission. Bruce Lee once said, "Absorb what is useful, reject what is useless, add what is essentially your own." In living by these words from my childhood hero, I came to see the distinction between therapy and training with pain showed less and less utility.

I'm happy to say that I remain good friends with the therapist I wound up partnering with—our subsequent parting of ways was strictly professional. Recommended to me by mutual acquaintances, Jim was exactly the sort of person I thought I needed. A climber himself, he held a doctorate in physical therapy from NAU and had a genuinely caring nature. And he was on board with my vision, so we teamed up. The idea was this: Athletes with injuries or pain experiences would come to us as patients. Jim would treat them, and then, when they were ready, these patients would become athletes again and I would train them. Jim had his role as therapist, I had mine as coach, and together we were like chocolate and peanut butter—perfect complements to each other.

One critical change began to occur as my understanding expanded. It was becoming more and more clear to me that the causal relationship between pain and tissue and biomechanics was not nearly as direct as many believe. I was fast gravitating toward an ecological approach to care, while Jim began moving more toward nuances of biomechanics. At the same time I lost faith in structuralism, Jim's structuralist views moved in the opposite direction, away from the mainstream. Specifically, Jim began using a treatment approach called *postural restoration*, which is like structuralism on steroids. Developed in the 1990s by Ron Hruska, a Nebraska-based physical therapist, postural restoration rests on the idea that although the body is fundamentally asymmetrical in structure, the more symmetrical one can make it, the better it functions. Practitioners of this discipline fuss over every measurable element of structural and functional balance, from the greatest to the smallest.

Even the teeth and eyes do not escape the attention of the therapist trained in postural restoration. Practitioners have been known to adjust a client's occlusion (bite) and prescribe prism glasses to patients, believing that these minute adjustments would rectify something in the nervous system that was presumed to be the cause of their pain. It wasn't my place to tell Jim how to practice, and I've never doubted his genuine care for people. However, the further I went in my career, the clearer it became to me that simple and practical coaching was the path forward.

Breathing is a major concern in postural restoration. It therefore became a major concern for some of the athletes Jim passed along to me after he'd finished treating them. My own take on breathing is that it's best not to overthink it. If you can breathe in your sleep, it's a safe bet you're doing it properly when you're awake as well. This put me in a tough spot when athletes asked me if I planned to continue the process of "fixing" their breathing that Jim had started with them. On the one hand, I didn't want to contradict Jim and confuse the athlete. On the other hand, I didn't want to just let the athlete keep worrying about something I didn't think they needed to worry about. Such notions can have lasting negative effects on people—not only prolonging their pain but exacerbating it through something called *biographical suspension*. This is essentially what it sounds like: When a form of treatment is difficult or impossible to complete (Can posture ever be fully restored?), it essentially puts the patient's life, or significant parts of it, on pause.

Jim and I knew we had gone as far as we could in our professional collaboration. He came to me one day and broke the news that he had decided to step away from Paragon, explaining that the gym setting was too "excitatory" for patients with persistent pain. I had to admit he had a point there, what with the high-energy music that filled the space at all hours. So we shook hands and parted ways. There were certainly no regrets on my side. And thus began my wholehearted commitment to a biopsychosocial approach.

A NEW PARTNERSHIP IN PAIN MANAGEMENT

I began to make changes at Paragon—tweaks, adjustments, and over-hauls that would, over time, evolve into Training as Treatment. The more I learned about the flaws in the structural model of athletic injury and about the new science of pain, the luckier I felt to be a trainer as opposed to any other type of provider. As a trainer, I am barred by law from diagnosing injuries and other medical conditions. I now see this limitation as a blessing, having learned that diagnosis often does more harm than good and should be done as sparingly as possible. I learned too that most of the common treatments for pain and nontraumatic injury are ineffective, but again, as a trainer, it was not my job to practice such treatments anyway. What *is* effective in managing athletic pain and injury, I discovered, is exercise, which is a trainer's medium. Also useful is good communication, and there are (thank goodness) no laws forbidding trainers from communicating constructively with athletes. Indeed, all good trainers take the inter-personal component of the job very seriously. I certainly did, but my immersion in the new science of pain had the effect of making me more conscious and strategic in my communication with athletes.

Much of what is communicated to individuals in a given envi-ronment comes from the environment itself. Before I even open up my mouth to greet a new athlete who's just walked through the door for the first time, that person has picked up certain messages from the space. And so as part of my new approach to communicating with athletes, I did a little redecorating at Paragon, removing things that conveyed the wrong message, however subtly. An expensive pair of laminated posters showing the locations of trigger points throughout the body came down off the walls. Nobody really knows what these sensitive spots of muscle fascia really are. But that's not what bothered me about the posters. At issue, rather, was that the posters insinuated their creators (Janet Travell and David Simons) *did* know what trigger points are. Consequently, having these posters displayed reinforced the broader misrepresentation that clinicians possess secret knowledge about musculoskeletal care, making athletes dependent on them for pain management.

Additionally, I removed a lot of books from the gym. I had all of Dr. Stuart McGill's works on back pain. Those disappeared along with several volumes on running biomechanics and any other book in my collection that might give athletes the impression that managing pain and injury is complicated, when in fact it's quite simple. I wasn't so naive as to think that a few small improvements in my facility's decor would unwind the programming that an athlete's mind has been subjected to for many years. But precisely because they had been steeped in the medicalization of athletic pain and injury, I felt the need to consistently communicate the Training as Treatment approach through every available medium.

Rearranging the furniture, so to speak, goes only so far to change the athlete-coach experience. Words matter more. Knowing this, I made psychology the next focus of my continual self-education. I read deeply in the field of cognitive behavioral therapy, a type of psychotherapy that uses structured dialogue to help individuals change unhelpful thoughts, emotions, and behaviors. Of particular interest to me was the practice of motivational interviewing, a technique whereby a therapist (or coach, as the case may be) uses strategic questioning to get patients (or athletes) to reflect deeply about what they want, why they want it, and how best to achieve it. The gym might be a less intuitive setting for this type of work, but motivational interviewing is every bit as relevant to athletic goals such as staying healthy, training productively, and improving performance as it is to more conventional therapeutic goals such as processing grief. When I discovered that my friend Buck Blankenship, a Flagstaff-based ultrarunner, was studying motivational interviewing in pursuit of a graduate degree in special education at NAU, I accepted his invitation to take part in virtual classes on the subject and subsequently brought him in to train new staff at Paragon in the technique.

AN ATHLETE-CENTRIC METHODOLOGY

Athletes often come to me for help because they feel they need me, and they might be right about that when they are just getting started, but I am determined to get each athlete to a place where they no longer need me to feel confident in working through a pain experience. To this end, I don't just practice Training as Treatment on athletes; I *teach* the process as we practice it together. Basketball coach Billy Donovan once said, "Believe in your system, and then sell it to your players." This is something every good coach does because every good coach knows their athletes get more out of any given training system when they understand and buy into it. The secret sauce in training is believing your training is the secret sauce.

Following an initial consultation with an athlete, I hand them a pad and a pen to take notes. I do this not because I'm too lazy to take my own notes but rather to signal to the athlete that I expect them to be an active participant in our partnership. It's a simple but effective way to start the process of cultivating pain self-efficacy—of teaching athletes how to catch their own fish, as the saying goes, instead of depending on me to put fish on their tables.

Another major goal of my communication with athletes is to get them to see the process of managing pain and injury as creative versus rote. Gone are the days when I went out of my way to show athletes how much I knew about the human body in general and about what was wrong with them specifically and how to "fix" them. Socrates said, "The only true wisdom is knowing you know nothing," and if this is true, then I'm a much wiser trainer than I used to be. I now realize that nobody knows exactly what pain is and what causes it or makes it go away in any particular instance. Furthermore, I know that following an open-ended, rule-guided trial-and-error process is the most effective way for any individual athlete to manage pain. In a sense, I've come full circle, returning to the intuitive way of operating that I adopted during my rough-and-tumble childhood and early adulthood, when I managed pain quite effectively in my own athletic pursuits not through academic knowledge but by following a process very much like the one I now call Training as Treatment.

Given their past experiences in medicine-centered pain and injury treatment, most athletes start their process of pain management focused on the end point. They want to know where treatment will end and training will resume. But in the Training as Treatment approach, there is no end point because you are always training. Athletes are accustomed to either/or thinking—they are either injured and in treatment or healthy and in training. Training as Treatment replaces this paradigm with an if/then alternative—if you are experiencing pain, then you're going to use the same tools that would be used for performance, adjusting the load, volume, velocity, and variety of movements as necessary. I tell athletes to think of their bodies as gardens and musculoskeletal care as gardening. A garden has no end point. As a gardener, you want your garden to flourish at all times. You never start or stop tending your garden—you just tend it in somewhat different ways in different seasons.

Having said all this, I will now add that if you were to visually compare how I worked with an athlete during my structuralist period to how I now use Training as Treatment, you might not see much difference—other than my gray hair. I still perform certain movement assessments, and of course, I still give athletes exercises to do. But how I communicate with athletes has changed radically. When I worked within the structuralist paradigm, I would start by telling the athlete what was wrong with their movements, describe the structural damage they've caused, and explain how to fix it. Today, you would hear me use very different language. Instead of describing an athlete's biomechanics as wrong or faulty, I explain how they are placing extra demand on certain tissues and propose ways of either reducing this demand, increasing the tolerance of the tissues, or modifying activity. My goal is always to help the athlete think in terms of working with what they've got rather than trying to move perfectly. When an athlete sheepishly admits to "cheating" in performing a certain movement (i.e., doing it "incorrectly" to make it easier), I will gently challenge their own language, suggesting that what they call *cheating* is more accurately labeled *kinematic cleverness*.

Not every athlete is immediately comfortable with me telling them "I don't know" in answer to questions like "What caused my pain?" or "How do I get rid of this pain and keep it from coming back?" In Chapter 4, I talked about how athletes (including me, at one time) are often willing participants in the theater that is the standard clinical experience. Many would rather hear dishonest certitude from a doctor, therapist, or trainer than honest uncertainty, at least for now. But the truth is that Training as Treatment just replaces one form of certainty with another. When I tell an athlete that I don't know the answer to their question, I don't stop there. The full answer is "I don't know, but we'll figure it out." Because it's true—we will. With Training as Treatment, we trust the process rather than our knowledge. Followed diligently, this process is certain to yield better long-term outcomes for the athlete than applying a one-size-fits-all treatment plan based on "knowledge" of which specific pathology an athlete represents and sticking to it no matter what. And the best part is, after working with me long enough to learn and understand the process, the athlete can practice it on their own in the future.

GETTING PAST THE PHYSICAL NATURE OF PAIN

The trickiest part of applying the biopsychosocial model of pain in the gym environment is the psychosocial part. I find it difficult to suggest to athletes that cognitive and emotional factors, such as expectations and stress, might be influencing their pain experience without being misinterpreted. Having internalized the dualistic notion that the body and the mind are completely separate, the one physical and the other nonphysical, many assume I'm suggesting that they're imagining their pain—or worse, that they have a screw loose. But that's not at all what I mean. What I mean is that pain is fundamentally an experience. It is not a physical phenomenon that produces a felt experience. Pain has no objective existence outside our experience. And like all experiences, pain is influenced by cognitive and emotional factors. This is true for everyone.

To a certain extent, I can manipulate psychological and social contributors to an athlete's pain experience without them even knowing it. I ask my clients lots of questions that may seem to have no relevance to the particular problem they want me to help them with. I do this partly because research has shown that physicians tend to get better treatment outcomes with patients when they establish and nurture personal connections with them. According to a study conducted by Stanford researchers and published in the *Journal of the American Medical Association* in 2020, five key practices are helpful in this regard: (1) taking time to prepare for each appointment, (2) listening intently, (3) learning what's most important to the patient and taking it seriously, (4) connecting with the patient's "story" (how they see their past, present, and future), and (5) paying attention to and validating the patient's emotions. I'm not a physician, but the coach-athlete relationship is very similar—I engage in all of the above practices for the athletes' clinical benefit, and it's clear they appreciate this human-to-human approach.

Where things get dicey sometimes is at that delicate point at which I shift from implicitly manipulating psychological and social factors to bringing these things out into the open. My favorite example is Stan (not his real name), a mountain biker who came to me complaining of low-back pain. He'd been dealing with the issue for seven years, and he was near the end of his rope. Prior to flying in from out of state to consult me, Stan had been to a succession of doctors and physical therapists and undergone the usual imaging tests with nothing to show for it beyond a consensus that his sacroiliac joint was messed up.

Knowing what I do about the biopsychosocial nature of low-back pain, I asked Stan what else was going on in his life—besides mountain biking, which he'd been taught to regard as the sole culprit vis-à-vis his "injury"—around the time of the pain's onset. He paused for a moment to rewind his memory seven years, shook his head, and answered that nothing noteworthy came to mind. I pressed a bit, and eventually Stan volunteered that, come to think of it, he had been going through a divorce then. Oh, and also, he was being investigated by the IRS. And he had recently contracted a venereal disease.

Now, it so happens that Stan was a psychologist. In light of this fact, I took a chance and suggested that perhaps the stressors he enumerated were contributing to his pain experience along with the physical stressors of riding his bike and whatever else. This did not go over well. Although he did not come right out and accuse me of insinuating his pain was imagined, I could tell by the look on Stan's face that he was having just as much trouble distinguishing between *psychological* and *imaginary* as my athletes who were not psychologists. He did not remain my client for very long before deciding to continue his search for a purely physical cure to what he considered to be a purely physical problem.

If that's as far as I got with most of my clients, I would be looking for work. But in the majority of cases, I'm happy to say, I do a better job of not getting ahead of myself on the psychosocial side of my practice and hence of not scaring folks off before they see its fruits. It helps that the failure rate in pain treatment—persistent pain in particular—is famously high. I've built my practice largely on last-chancers—athletes and others whom medical doctors and physical therapists have been unable to help. A number of these professionals now refer these cases to me, regarding me as a clinician of last resort, though it is my opinion that most of them would be better off coming to me, or someone like me, first.

DON'T SETTLE FOR PERMANENT PAIN

A typical case is Elano, who came to me as a 32-year-old police officer facing early retirement from the local police force due to knee pain. A competitive tennis player and an all-around superfit dude, Elano had torn an anterior cruciate ligament (ACL) working out. After surgery, he entered physical therapy, where he remained for two years—far longer than should have been necessary for someone in his situation. The problem was not that he couldn't use the leg—he got most of his range of motion and a lot of his strength back in those two years—but that it still hurt like hell to do anything strenuous like, say, the work of a police officer! Per usual, it was only when Elano was on the brink of being judged a lost cause that he was finally referred to me.

The reason therapy had failed Elano was twofold. First, the exercises he was given were specific to his injury, not to him. Each person's pain experience is unique. This is why managing pain—whether after knee surgery or at any other time—requires ongoing experimentation, adaptation, and learning on the go. Eliminating pain as a barrier to full activity requires that you do the closest thing to normal activity that you can without making the pain worse. The aim is to perform movements that work around and toward the pain, gradually increasing loads and specificity as the pain barrier recedes. Elano's therapists did not do this.

The second reason Elano didn't get much benefit from physical therapy was that the therapists were too pain avoidant and leaned on primarily passive tools, such as massage, dry needling, stretching, and so on. Many clinicians view all significant pain as a red flag indicating aggravation of underlying damage. But after two years of recovery, there could not have been much tissue damage left in Elano's knee, so his pain wasn't necessarily a cue to back off. Knowing this, I started *training* him, giving him movements that were specific to the tasks he used to perform on his beat and on the tennis court, with loading he could tolerate. Of course, we remained respectful of his pain, but we were not fearful. In the beginning, he experienced a good bit of pain, but I assured him he wasn't harming himself, and he trusted me. Within six months, Elano was fully recovered and ready for duty, and when I last heard from him, his tennis game was stronger than ever.

I can't tell you how satisfying it is to help people in this way. But I can only help so many. Even though the whole point of Training as Treatment is to empower athletes to manage their own pain, this teaching process has required one-on-one interaction. We need a lot more trainers and physical therapists to accept and master the same approach, and we need a lot more doctors to accept it as well and begin to refer people with nontraumatic musculoskeletal pain and injuries to practitioners like me—not as a last resort but as a first step. Progress in this direction has been frustratingly slow, however, for a couple of reasons.

EVANGELIZING A NEW METHOD
OF PAIN MANAGEMENT

In January 2017, I invited Greg Lehman to lead a two-day clinic called Reconciling Biomechanics with Pain Science here in Flagstaff. It was at this event that I realized what we were up against in pursuing our shared mission to demedicalize musculoskeletal care. Greg is a skillful presenter who has led iterations of the same clinic dozens of times all over the map. He did a bang-up job at the event I hosted for him, but his message was mostly lost on the 40-ish clinicians and roughly half-dozen trainers (and one yogi, my friend Jules, from whose lips I first heard Greg Lehman's name) who attended.

He kicked off day one by asking audience members—most of them MDs, PTs, and PhDs—to identify musculoskeletal patholo-gies that, in their opinion, required specific treatment, meaning a protocol tailored to that particular injury or condition. Hands were confidently raised and pathologies assuredly named ("supraspinatus tendinopathy" is the one I remember). Greg then proceeded to coldly invalidate their respective treatment protocols one by one. In each case, Greg cited research demonstrating that the specific treatment for the named pathology was ineffective. Cumulatively, these mer-cilessly dispassionate refutations made the point that specific treat-ment protocols are not the proper way to address such pathologies, and even the diagnosis itself has little utility. All the clinician really needs to know, he intimated, is "where it hurts."

On day two, having said enough about the wrong way to address pain and dysfunction, Greg talked about what he believes is the right way, or at least the best way available to us today. In his practice, diag-nosis is eschewed on the grounds that it serves no practical purpose and also tends to negatively affect the expectations of the person being diagnosed. Instead of naming the problem causing the person's pain, he focuses on the person first, pain second, and biomechanics last. Treatment consists almost entirely of symptom modification—helping the person do more with less pain—which is achieved mainly through strength training and other exercise. Along the way, Greg is careful to demonstrate his expertise only to the extent that is necessary to gain and preserve the person's trust and never for the sake of asserting dominance in the clinical relationship. And he listens more than he talks.

As Greg described his biopsychosocial approach to managing pain, I nodded along, recognizing all the key elements of the Training as Treatment approach I practice at Paragon Athletics. It all made so much sense that I failed to notice the blank stares on the faces around me. When the clinic wrapped up, I went around the room asking the attendees what they thought, expecting their excitement to match my own. Almost without exception, these highly trained professionals either hadn't understood what they'd heard from Greg or understood all too well but refused to accept it.

A REVOLUTION IN PAIN MANAGEMENT

I want to live in a world where athletes do not shift from sports training to medical treatment when experiencing pain associated with nontraumatic musculoskeletal injuries but instead train through it either with the help of a coach, trainer, or biopsychosocial-informed clinician or on their own. What bugs me is that I'm not sure I will live long enough to see this world. Progress toward demedicalized pain management has been a lot slower than, in my naivete, I expected it to be when I first recognized the need for it. But there has been some progress. For example, in 2018, the American Physical Therapy Association and the National Athletic Trainers Association announced a new collaborative relationship. More symbolic than substantive, the creation of a direct communication channel between organizations with *therapy* and *training* in their respective names is a step in the right direction. In recent years, I've also seen slow growth in the number of individual scientists, doctors, and other high-level clinicians who appear to take me seriously, are open to answering my many questions, and seem to be paying attention to what I'm doing at Paragon. Still, the major impediments to the full-scale revolution that's warranted—namely, money and professional self-interest—remain in place.

Imagine what it was like for carriage builders when the automobile revolution occurred in the early 20th century. That's kind of what it's like for clinicians who treat activity-related pain and injury today. Any clinician who doesn't offer training as a tool to manage these things is poorly positioned to help athletes in the way the new pain science indicates is best. The right thing to do in this situation is to either acquire this tool or refer would-be patients to clinicians who do offer training. But instead, most clinicians are staying the course, continuing to treat patients as though the structural model of injury hasn't been scientifically invalidated and the biopsychosocial model doesn't exist.

It often happens in science that when a prevailing theory or model's predictions fail, its proponents, loath to abandon it, try to patch it up instead. Ptolemy's model of the solar system is the quintessential example of this phenomenon. Not understanding the nature of gravity, the ancient Alexandrian astronomer made his model increasingly complex in reaction to its failure to accurately predict planetary motions. In a similar fashion, the structural model of pain has become increasingly esoteric as its proponents scramble to assimilate experimental findings that challenge its legitimacy.

Recently, I witnessed an online forum debate among scientists concerning the validity of the term *nociplastic*, which refers to pain that lacks an underlying structural source. It went on for nearly a week, back and forth, around and around. I refrained from chiming in, but if I had, my contribution would have been this: *Who cares?*

I'm not suggesting that terminology doesn't matter—everyone knows that defining terms in science and philosophy is integral to the process. But on the application side of things, fussing over semantics loses the forest for the trees, and in this instance, I saw the semantic nitpicking as emblematic of a larger effort to ensure that clinical pain management is too complex for pragmatists like me to competently practice. And the truth, once again, is that effective management of pain is simple, if not always easy.

THE REAL EXPERT ON YOUR PAIN

These days, more and more clinicians refer to themselves as pain experts or specialists. But the real pain expert is *you*. If you know how to put on a sweater when you feel chilly, you know how to manage pain. The only difference is that the medical establishment has made you believe you don't know how to manage pain, which is true to the extent that accepting this doctrine has caused you to forget some of what you used to know. But this kind of knowledge is never really lost. It's just buried under a bunch of crap.

I'm not saying pain specialists shouldn't exist. There are certain scenarios that demand someone who understands more complex pain processes. For the lion's share of pain experiences, however, this level of expertise is probably not necessary. Clinicians who hope to help as many people—athletes and nonathletes—as possible should be focused on simplifying pain management, not on doing the opposite for the sake of job security, as too many do.

A good example of unnecessary complexification in pain and injury treatment involves newer brain-centered methods of restoring function after ACL surgery. It's been shown by fMRI that there are changes in the brain (specifically the motor cortex) that occur after an ACL repair. To address this problem, scientists and clinicians have developed protocols for zapping the brain with transcranial electromagnetic energy and activating the quadriceps in specific ways intended to restore "corticospinal excitability." The problem with all of this is not so much that it doesn't work as that it doesn't work as well, as cheaply, and as efficiently as good training, as our friend Elano can vouch. Remember, the more sciency way to do something is not always the better way.

Could Elano have found his way back to the police force and the tennis court without my help? Maybe, maybe not. But if—heaven forbid—he should ever blow out the other knee, I think he just might be able to train his way back to 100 percent on his own based on what he learned (and relearned) about pain in our time together. And that's the point. As I said before, it's not a huge stretch to say that my job, as I see it, is to put myself out of a job.

Admittedly, it's not a job I will ever complete. Athletes do sometimes need expert help in managing pain and always will. The question is, Where do they go for that help? You can answer this question just by thinking about where you have gone in the past. Has it ever even crossed your mind to call a trainer first? Probably not, for two reasons. One is that athletes are taught to seek help from doctors and physical therapists when they're in pain. The other is that very few trainers practice Training as Treatment or anything like it. I don't foresee doctors conceding anytime soon that athletes with nontraumatic musculoskeletal injuries don't belong in their offices. Nor am I holding out hope that the physical therapy profession will get fully on board with Training as Treatment. Given this reality, if the changes I want to see happen are actually going to happen in my lifetime, we need to make them happen without expecting much help from members of the medical establishment.

That's right, I said *we*. Sometimes change starts at home—or in this case, in the gym. It's my hope that *Pain and Performance* will not only help individual athletes self-manage athletic pain and injury but also start a movement. By empowering athletes like you to manage pain on your own or with the help of coaches and trainers, I seek to create a demand for a new generation of trainers and clinicians who base their practice on good scientific evidence and a biopsychosocial model of pain. In a Training as Treatment environment, the professional's primary "treatment" tools are training and coaching according to the needs of the individual athlete. Your part in this movement is simple: keep reading.

THE NEW SCIENCE OF PAIN

In 2019, I worked briefly with Jessica, an active, outdoorsy woman in her 30s who held a job as a nurse practitioner on a Native American reservation. Unlike most of the athletes I coach, who are dealing with a recent or somewhat recent injury that is really bugging them, Jessica wanted help for hip pain that had been affecting her since she was injured in a car wreck when she was 15 years old. Except for bicycling, the lingering discomfort didn't stop her from doing most of the stuff she wanted to do, which is more than many persistent pain sufferers can say.

Pain that you're used to is still pain, though, and Jessica sought me out for a reason. Simply put, she wanted more for herself. Despite the many specialists she'd seen and the many diagnostics that had been performed, nothing had ever been found that could explain her pain. As far as the specialists were concerned, this meant the pain couldn't be fixed (if it existed at all). But Jessica believed things could get better for her, and I agreed.

In addition to being a medical professional, Jessica is a person with whom I have a good rapport. So we had quite a few in-depth discussions about pain, and I felt comfortable using more technical jargon with her than I do with most of my clients. If I remember correctly, it was during our second session that, acting on a hunch, I invited Jessica to name a specific movement that never failed to provoke pain in her hip. Without hesitation, she picked the split squat, which entails squatting toward the floor from a lunge position, like a quarterback taking a knee at the end of a football game. I then asked Jessica to perform the movement while I filmed it with an iPad, and sure enough, it hurt. Next, I suggested that she perform the provocative movement while watching the video I had just recorded. This may seem like an arbitrary experiment, but I assure you I wouldn't be arbitrary with anyone's pain experience or health. This was purely a case of Jessica and me being curious.

"Huh, that's weird," she said.

"What's weird?" I asked.

"No pain."

Before you run off and film yourself doing something that hurts, understand the full context. The sudden disappearance of Jessica's hip pain was not accidental, but it wasn't evidence of a "cure" either. All I'd done was deflect her attention in a way that caused her nervous system to do something other than the usual thing when she performed a split squat. I should also point out that although I did have a hunch that the technique I tried on Jessica might do exactly what it did, I wasn't exactly expecting it to work. For this very reason, I wouldn't have tried it on an athlete who was more desperate for relief from their pain. And I was careful to present the exercise to her as an experiment, nothing more.

Unfortunately, the COVID-19 pandemic struck not long after this session took place, so Jessica and I weren't able to finish the process we'd started together. But that one weird moment alone made a big difference for her. When I say it wasn't a cure, I mean just that—she still had hip pain. What changed was her perspective on her pain experience. The video trick I tried on Jessica challenged her assumptions and showed her what was possible. She saw that she could change her pain, and this new sense of control was empowering. When I last heard from Jessica, she'd gotten back into cycling, not without pain, but without fear of imminent discomfort. It's a terrific example of how game-changing it can be to base our response to pain on cutting-edge pain science—with its biological, psychological, and social dimensions—rather than on the outmoded idea that pain and injury are coextensive.

The specific piece of cutting-edge pain science I had in mind when I proposed my little experiment to Jessica was *cortical smudging*, which is the brain's ability to alter the way it represents a given part of the body to the conscious mind. A broken bone takes weeks to heal no matter what, but the brain can instantaneously change its motorsensory map of the right hip or any other piece of anatomy in response to a particular stimulus. But to be completely candid, I couldn't say whether it was this mechanism or a different one that caused the change, and neither could anyone else.

As with many fields of science, the more we learn about pain, the more we realize how much we don't know. Nevertheless, what scientists have learned about pain is useful in helping athletes navigate the experience of it, as my story about Jessica illustrates. Personally, I find pain science to be utterly fascinating, and I hope to spark your curiosity around the topic. But the true purpose of the following brief tour of pain science is to empower you in the same way Jessica was empowered by what she learned. Understanding pain better will alter your relationship with it in a way that gives you greater control and confidence in your future experiences with it.

THE BRAIN'S ROLE IN PAIN

By its very nature, pain gets people's attention. It's not surprising, then, that philosophers and scientists have been theorizing about pain for as long as there have been philosophers and scientists.

The influential 17th-century French thinker René Descartes is widely credited with having developed the first modern scientific theory of pain, which he described in his book *Treatise of Man*, published posthumously in 1664. What made Descartes's explanation both modern and scientific was that unlike prior attempts to explain pain, it located the pain experience inside the brain. Earlier thinkers had taken it for granted that if your foot hurt, the pain was in your foot.

In his treatise, Descartes illustrated his take on pain with an example involving foot pain. A man is shown sitting with his left foot a bit too close to an open fire. Heat particles from the fire touch the skin and tug on nerve endings. This tugging effect travels all the way to the brain, causing valves to open at the point where the nerve fibers originate and communicating the painful stimulus to the man's conscious mind. "Animal spirits" then travel through the nerve fibers from the brain back to the foot, which moves away from the flame to escape the painful stimulus. This is known as the Cartesian pain model.

A theory can be both a step forward for science and wrong. Newtonian physics was a huge improvement on the primitive explanations of motion it replaced, and to this day it remains useful for simple construction projects. But if we try to apply Newtonian physics to explain the mysteries of the universe, we are going to end up woefully off course. The same is true of Descartes's theory of pain. What it gets right is that pain happens in the mind, not the body. What it gets wrong, however, is the proposition that noxious stimuli from "pain fibers" (nociceptors) were all that was required to "complete the circuit" and produce the experience of pain. We now have a much better understanding of the complexity of pain.

The next step toward this better understanding came in 1965, when Canadian psychologist Ronald Melzack and British neuroscientist Patrick Wall introduced the gate control theory of pain. Building on then recent advances in neuroanatomy, this theory replaced

Descartes's valves with a gating mechanism in the spinal column that either allows pain signals to pass through or inhibits them based on the specific type of nerve fiber carrying them.

The key advantage of gate control theory over the Cartesian pain model is that it is able to account for psychological and social influences on pain perception, such as stress and fear. As we saw in the burnt foot illustration, Descartes viewed the brain as a slave to the body where pain is concerned. But everyone knows from lived experience that mental states and traits factor into pain as well. In a 1968 paper, Melzack offered the well-known example of soldiers reporting little or no pain after being grievously wounded in battle and proposed that the special cognitive state that soldiers experience in such circumstances might exert an inhibitory effect on pain gates that is stronger than nociceptive signals traveling from the site of injury to the brain, keeping the gates shut. Nevertheless, gate control theory is fundamentally physiological in nature and tends to regard the actual experience of pain as an epiphenomenon rather than as the main story.

In this respect, gate control theory was wholly consistent with other prevailing biomedical theories, models, and concepts of its time, none of which looked at things from the patient's (for lack of a better word) point of view. American psychiatrist George Engel took issue with this bias. While he recognized the value of learning about how the body functions in both healthy and diseased states, he believed that patients' health interests would be better served if clinicians took psychological and social influences on health as seriously as they took biological influences. In the seminal 1977 paper in which he introduced the biopsychosocial model, Engel wrote,

> The boundaries between health and disease, between well and sick,
> are far from clear, and will never be clear, for they are diffused by

cultural, social, and psychological considerations. The traditional biomedical view, that biological indices are the ultimate criteria defining disease, leads to the present paradox that some people with positive laboratory findings are told they are in need of treatment when in fact they are feeling quite well, while others feeling sick are assured that they are well; that is, they have no "disease." A biopsychosocial model which includes the illness as well as the patient would encompass both circumstances.

The biopsychosocial model is not specific to pain, but pain treatment has been one of its main applications since the model's introduction. Dozens of experiments have lent empirical support to Engel's insight. A 2008 study conducted by an interdisciplinary team of Oxford University scientists, for example, found that subjects who were devout Catholics experienced less pain than nonreligious subjects and exhibited increased activation in a brain area known to be involved in pain modulation when viewing an image of the Virgin Mary while being subjected to a painful stimulus, validating the biopsychosocial view that pain is a social construct.

Treatments based on the biopsychosocial model have been shown repeatedly to yield better results than those based on the biomedical model. A 2018 paper in the *British Medical Journal* reported that Australian ethnic minorities with chronic pain were more likely to adhere to physiotherapy treatment and experienced a greater reduction in pain and a larger increase in function when the program was culturally adapted for them. Nothing physical was different between this program and a standard program used with subjects in a control group; only the messaging differed.

I don't want to give you the impression that current advancements in pain science are happening entirely on the psychological and social side and not at all on the side of biology. On the contrary, research into the physiological underpinnings of pain continues to progress at a rapid pace. Nor do I want to give you the impression that the psycho-social and biological dimensions of pain are separate. One of the most exciting things that's happening in pain science today is that research-ers from disparate fields are working together and communicating with one another, the result of which is an understanding of pain that isn't as one-sided as past conceptualizations of the phenomenon. The Oxford study I mentioned is a great example. It was performed by a combination of neuroscientists, philosophers, psychologists, and theologians, and the results informed our understanding of the bio-logical, psychological, and social dimensions of pain.

Lastly, I would be remiss if I failed to acknowledge that many other theories and models of pain exist today. These include Loeser's onion model, the neuromatrix model, and the threat model. The very existence of so many competing pain theories is evidence of the fact that we still have a lot to learn on the topic, a reality that is likely to persist for a very long time to come. And that's OK. As athletes, we don't need to know precisely what pain is. However, we do need to know how to work with it. In this regard, there are four fundamental truths about pain that are reconfirmed by each new advancement in pain science and have special practical relevance to athletes. They are as follows:

1. Pain is mysterious.
2. Pain is information.
3. Pain is individual.
4. Pain is controllable.

Let's briefly explore each of these truths with a special focus on what they mean for you as an athlete who's interested in successful self-management of pain and injury.

PAIN IS MYSTERIOUS

When I was 19 years old, I spent some time studying epistemology at a Swiss commune. It sounds like the setup for a joke, but it's true. Epistemology is a branch of philosophy that deals with knowledge. One of the things I learned during this period is that there's a difference between *unknown* and *unknowable*. An unknown is essentially a question that we don't have an answer to yet. An unknowable is a question that we know we will never be able to answer.

Ironically, one of the chief lessons that recent advances in pain science have taught us is that some things about it are unknowable. For example, we know that we will never know precisely what causes pain. Suppose you're walking barefoot and you step on a thumbtack and feel pain. In this scenario, it might seem obvious that the tack caused your pain, but if this were true, then stepping on a tack would *always* cause pain, and we know from research that there is no single event that causes pain invariably.

My most unforgettable experience of pain's fathomless complexity involved Janice (not her real name), an elite runner who'd been unable to compete for more than two years when I started working with her. Throughout this tortuous ordeal, Janice had been seen by a physical therapist and had extensive imaging done on her foot, leg, hip, and back, for her pain was migratory and never centered in one location for very long. Although none of her images showed anything out of the ordinary, Janice had nevertheless received many musculoskeletal diagnoses and was also told her gait was causing her pain. Bear in mind this is a professional athlete.

After a few months of Training as Treatment, she was able to begin competing again, rising all the way back to the world stage. Sadly, after experiencing pain during one of her competitions, Janice made a desperate decision to return to her therapist, who claimed her hip needed to be adjusted in order for her to run "correctly."

Sometime later, Janice texted me a photo of her swollen foot, captioned, "I don't think this is all in my head."

This was a punch to the gut. I thought back through our conversations and could not figure out for the life of me how this was what she came away with. Janice seemed to feel vindicated by her latest diagnosis—a bone stress reaction—but the images were inconclusive, and she had none of the major risk factors linked with this type of injury (namely, sudden changes in diet or training and prior bone injuries). Although I never told Janice her pain was all in her head, I had told her I believed her pain was not caused primarily by structural damage to her foot, leg, hip, or back, and I still believe this. A more likely diagnosis, in my opinion, was complex regional pain syndrome, whose sufferers often experience pain, swelling, and even discoloration with no mechanical causes to be found. But this does not mean the pain is all in their heads. It's just weird.

"Hold on a second," you say. "If pain is a sensation alone, and sensations are created by the brain, can we at least identify a specific brain state that is associated with the experience of pain?" Nope! Research has revealed that there is no single brain state associated with the experience of pain. While it is true that sensations are rooted in the brain, the brain exhibits a quality called *degeneracy*, which simply means that multiple brain states can produce the same sensation. Hence it is inaccurate to state that any particular brain state is the cause of a given pain experience. As leading pain researcher Lorimer Moseley has written, "The biology of pain is never really straightforward, even when it appears to be."

The fact that pain is irreducibly mysterious and will never be fully understood is actually good news because it means you can never say never with pain. If pain were something we understood entirely—if it obeyed known laws with 100 percent consistency and were therefore fully predictable—then you would be doomed to experience pain whenever science said that pain was inevitable. The fact that pain is not rigidly mechanistic—not something that always occurs when a particular thing happens to or within your body—gives you power in your relationship with pain. Pain is mercurial, but for this very reason, you need not be a slave to it.

PAIN IS INFORMATION

Despite the fact that pain is not fully knowable, it's not a *complete* mystery. Seldom, if ever, is the manifestation of pain truly arbitrary, happening for no reason at all. Pain does behave with some consistency, which makes it fairly predictable and hence preventable and treatable to a certain degree. For example, you can avoid much of the pain you'd undoubtedly experience in your legs after running down a mountain by practicing downhill running for a few weeks before attempting the challenge. Likewise, you can also predictably overcome the pain of tennis elbow or any other so-called overuse injury by following the Training as Treatment process described in Chapter 7.

Any phenomenon that exhibits identifiable patterns in its behavior contains information, and this is true of pain. One of the keys to managing pain effectively as an athlete is finding the information in it and putting it to use. Tendon expert Ebonie Rio has observed that ruptures of the Achilles tendon occur far more often in athletes who experienced little or no pain in the tendon beforehand than in athletes who have significant Achilles pain. This is the opposite of what most people would expect, but the explanation makes perfect sense: Achilles pain motivates athletes to avoid overstressing the tendon. This is a good example of finding and putting to use the information contained in pain.

Unsurprisingly, the most successful athletes tend to mine the most information from pain, using it not only to avoid overdoing it in workouts but also to learn about their bodies' limits and evolve personalized approaches to training that minimize pain-induced disruptions to their progress. When I encounter an athlete who previously lost a lot of training days to injury but doesn't anymore, I can assume this is an athlete who has learned a lot from pain.

Professional ultrarunner Jared Hazen is one such athlete. A true prodigy, Jared was winning major trail races while still in high school. He was also logging 150- to 170-mile weeks routinely—and they weren't exactly flat miles. Jared's youth allowed him to get away with this punishing regimen for a while, but in 2017, he suffered not one but two stress fractures. I started working with him the following year, when he was dealing with yet another injury—a pesky case of osteitis pubis, or inflammation in the pubic bone. In the several years that have passed since then, Jared has gotten a lot better at keeping injuries from getting out of hand, and I believe the biggest reason is that he's learned from pain.

The process began when he won the 2018 JFK 50K after following a conservative training plan that was designed for the sole purpose of ensuring he reached the start line healthy. It was an eye-opening lesson and one he's carried forward. The Jared Hazen of today understands his limits and respects them. He's found a volume sweet spot around 120 miles per week, where he hangs out until just a few weeks before a race, at which point he'll bang out a few heavier weeks, but only if his body feels up to it. When he does experience warning signals, he no longer ignores and tries to push through them or panics and stops running altogether, switching into treatment mode. Instead, he modifies his training after taking a day or two off and either calls me or starts doing some of the exercises I've taught him in the past. Although still relatively young, Jared is experienced enough now that he seldom experiences an issue he hasn't dealt with before, so he knows what to do, or at least how to figure out what to do. The results speak for themselves. When Jared developed plantar fasciitis—another notoriously challenging running injury—toward the end of 2020, he reduced his running and shifted over to flat routes, replacing the running he was missing with cross-training. Thanks to this combination of self-efficacy and variation, he was back to full training within five weeks.

So yes, pain is a valuable teacher. It isn't always a reliable information source, however, and it's good to keep this in mind in your dealings with it. A relatively new theory of consciousness called *predictive processing* proposes that our perceptions—including our pain perception—are based largely on expectations and not so much on what is actually happening. And our expectations, in turn, are based on past experiences, which our brains use to create models of reality that make the world more predictable. This theory helps us understand why pain often manifests in the absence of structural damage to the body and why it often persists long after healing is complete in cases when it is initially linked to structural damage. It also makes sense of why expectancy violations, like the video trick I tried on Jessica, can be powerful tools for managing pain.

The upshot of all this is that it's best to approach your pain experiences with a healthy degree of skepticism and remain open to the possibility that the message they seem to be sending you is misleading. In particular, ask yourself, "Does this movement hurt because it's really not a good idea right now or because I fear or expect that I'm hurting myself by doing it?" To be clear, in expressing this caveat, I'm not dismissing the information pain offers. I'm just suggesting that like a lot of information sources, it is open to interpretation. Indeed, getting better at interpreting pain and knowing when it's misleading you is a core part of the process.

PAIN IS INDIVIDUAL

People with red hair have long been known to experience pain differently than people with other hair colors. Specifically, research has shown that redheads tend to be more sensitive to certain types of pain yet often have higher pain tolerances. Many also respond differently to pain medications. The reason has to do with a gene variant that regulates both hair color and certain hormones that affect pain perception.

This is one illustration of the many reasons pain is experienced differently among individuals. It happens to be a biological example, but a number of psychological and social factors are known to affect individual pain experience as well. Among these is familiarity. The more times you experience a particular type of pain, the more your relationship with it will evolve. This was shown in a widely reported 2019 study by Israeli researchers in which strength athletes, endurance athletes, and nonathlete controls were subjected to different pain stimuli. The key finding was that while both types of athletes were less sensitive to pain than nonathletes, strength athletes were less sensitive to pain than endurance athletes, who in turn had higher pain tolerances. The authors of this study concluded that these differences in pain experience likely represented adaptive responses to training and competition. In other words, the athletes had gotten good at dealing with the particular sort of pain their sport had accustomed them to, or the context of the experience had changed over time.

Beliefs are another important psychological influence on individual pain experience. Certain types of beliefs tend to exacerbate pain, while others have the opposite effect. Among the most cited studies on the effect of beliefs on individual pain experiences was one conducted by a team of Swiss researchers headed by Achim Elfering of the University of Bern and published in the *Scandinavian Journal of Work and Environmental Health* in 2009. In it, 264 adults experiencing low-back pain completed questionnaires concerning their beliefs about pain and were subsequently monitored for an entire year. Those who believed that current pain made future pain inevitable were found to have experienced higher levels of pain during the study period, as were those who believed that activities involving the use of the back were risky and should be avoided.

It's worth pointing out that beliefs are alterable, as are many of the other factors that influence individual pain experiences. An important implication of this fact is that pain experiences vary not only among individuals but also within individuals over time. I was reminded of this recently when I developed pain in my left shoulder—the first problem of this sort I'd experienced since over-coming my yearlong struggle with pain in my right shoulder back in 2005. Its onset, intensity, and behavior were very similar to that prior episode, but everything else about the experience was different, because I was different.

I first felt this new pain while reaching overhead with my left arm for a grip during a training climb—hardly a strain for someone who at times has been able to do multiple one-arm pull-ups. Over the ensuing days and weeks, the pain waxed and waned and moved around with no discernible cause-effect pattern. In all these respects, it reminded me of my last bout of shoulder pain. But unlike that experience, I felt no need to seek a diagnosis, identify the pain's cause, or stop training and climbing. In fact, I did one of my hardest workouts on the very day when the pain was at its worst. During the workout, I second-guessed my decision, but at the same time, I reminded myself that making mistakes is part of the process, and I wasn't really concerned about setting myself back in a serious way. Sure enough, the next day, the shoulder felt better than it had in weeks.

Overall, I felt confident in my ability to muddle through the process on my own and accepted that there was no way I could know in advance how it would play out. I took comfort as well in recognizing that allostatic load was a likely contributor to the pain experience, just as it had been with my right shoulder but without my awareness. In this case, the stress came from the COVID-19 pandemic, which hit

Paragon Athletics hard, requiring a rapid retooling of the business. But I knew the stress I was under wouldn't last forever and that its eventual dissipation would likely reduce my pain, and I was right.

The lesson here is that because pain is individual, each and every athlete has the power to change how they experience pain by changing themselves. Which brings us to the last of our four key truths about pain.

PAIN IS MANAGEABLE

Some of the coolest pain studies have been designed and carried out by Lorimer Moseley, who was previously mentioned. One of my favorite studies involved 10 subjects suffering from chronic pain in their dominant right hand. Moseley asked each subject to perform a sequence of standardized hand movements at a controlled pace and intensity. These movements were expected to cause pain and swelling in the hand, and the subjects had to repeat them on four separate occasions. On one occasion, the subjects did not look at their hand while performing the movements; on another (the actual order of the four conditions was randomized), they performed them while looking at their hand through binoculars without magnification; on a third occasion, the binoculars were set to make their hand look two times larger than normal while they used it; and in the remaining trial, the binoculars did the opposite, making their hand look two times smaller.

As expected, the subjects experienced an increase in pain and swelling in all four conditions, but there were significant differences among the four. On average, subjective pain ratings increased by 41 points on a 100-point scale when the hand was magnified, compared to just 19 points when the hand was made to look smaller. Pain levels also took the longest to return to baseline after the magnification trial, and if that wasn't enough, this same condition produced a measurably greater increase in swelling.

When these findings were published in 2008, they had both theoretical and clinical repercussions. On the theoretical side, they challenged science's understanding of the relationship between pain and body image, while on the clinical side, they suggested a potential new tool for pain treatment. At the most basic level, the discovery that how we see ourselves affects our pain experience demonstrated that pain is more controllable than most people think.

By the way, it's no coincidence that Lorimer Moseley thought up this experiment. When Moseley was fresh out of physiotherapy school, he decided to take a hitchhiking tour through Australia's South Coast. The first driver to offer him a lift was an eccentric gentleman with a prosthetic leg. At one point during the ride, this person began screaming in pain, his hands clenching the steering wheel so tightly the knuckles turned white. Powerless to help him, Moseley looked on in paralytic horror as the agonized driver fished around for and eventually found a screwdriver, handed it to Moseley, and asked him to jab it into a hole in the foot of the prosthetic. The instant he did so, the driver—who also demanded that Moseley move his head out of the way as he undertook the procedure so he could *see* the implement go into the hole, which had been helpfully prelabeled "Right Here"—stopped screaming and exhaled in relief as his hands relaxed.

When Moseley tells this story, he draws attention to two key lessons it teaches us. One is the obvious point that pain must be a brain-centered, top-down phenomenon if it can be felt "in" an appendage that doesn't belong to the person feeling it. The other lesson has to do with the controllability of pain. Somehow, this person figured out that if someone else inserted a screwdriver into a hole in the foot of his prosthetic *and* he watched it happen, his phantom limb pain would vanish. This story also underscores the fact that the true expert on any given pain experience is the person experiencing it. Although the one-legged driver needed others' help to control his pain, no one other than him could have come up with the solution he did.

Phantom limb pain is regarded as nociplastic, a catchall category for pain that doesn't fit within the main categories of nociceptive (pain influenced by inflammation or tissue damage) or neuropathic (pain linked to nerve damage). By its nature, nociplastic pain responds to a wider range of control measures than the other types, which account for virtually all sport-related pain experiences. Still, athletes have significant control—and oftentimes more control than they realize—over the types of pain they commonly encounter in training. Recognizing this control is the first step toward wielding it.

USING EXERCISE TO ADDRESS THE PHENOMENON OF PAIN

The civilization of ancient Egypt was known for many impressive innovations, including a host of discoveries and advances in the field of astronomy. Egyptian astronomers were able to use celestial measurements to create calendars, clocks, and time standards that were so accurate we still use them today with only the tiniest of modifications. Their knowledge of the stars was put to many practical uses, among which was predicting the seasons and thereby facilitating agricultural productivity. Remarkably, they did all of this without actually knowing what stars were!

As this example shows, it is not always necessary to fully understand a phenomenon to make practical use of it. This is very much the case with pain. In this chapter, I have taken pains (so to speak) to underscore the fact that there is much we don't know about pain. But of all the things we do know, none has firmer scientific backing than pain's responsiveness to exercise. Chronic low-back pain (CLBP), for example, is the leading cause of disability worldwide, and exercise is recognized as the most effective treatment for the condition. But guess what: Scientists cannot explain how exercise mitigates low-back pain!

In addition to knowing a lot about celestial movements, the ancient Egyptians certainly knew—intuitively, at least—that exercise was good medicine for pain, as have all humans for as long as our species has existed. Does this mean science has nothing to contribute? I wouldn't go that far. Consider the case of my father-in-law, Jim, a real-life cowboy who herds cattle on horseback and wears the whole hat-boots-and-belt-buckle getup. A number of years ago, Jim fell off a horse and injured his shoulder. Like any good cowboy, he didn't seek medical treatment for the problem but instead rehabilitated the shoulder on his own, engaging in a trial-and-error process of using it as much as he could without pushing to the point of increasing his pain level and gradually working his way back to full function.

The thing is, this process took 10 years. So when Jim hurt the shoulder again in a metal-forging accident, he came to me. I explained to him that I would guide him through a process that was similar to the one he'd used to overcome the previous injury but with a bit more pain science behind it. Within three months, Jim was mostly pain-free and back to full strength. Point being, yes, pain science does have a practical role to play in shaping how exercise is used in pain management. My name for the part-scientific, part-learn-by-doing method I used to help my father-in-law is—as you know—Training as Treatment, and in the next chapter, at long last, I will explain everything you need to know to start practicing it.

THE MOVEMENT DRUG

In March 2016, my coauthor, Matt, felt a sudden jolt of pain in his left knee while running a marathon. Just over a mile away from the finish line when it happened, he toughed out the remaining distance despite his discomfort and despite the fact that he was scheduled to compete in a 50-mile ultramarathon two weeks later. For the next 11 days, Matt restricted himself to nonimpact cross-training, hoping to preserve his fitness while allowing whatever damage he'd done to heal.

Two days before the 50-miler, Matt tested the knee with an easy jog. Alas, it hurt from the very first step and got worse with each subsequent step, so he bailed after 10 demoralizing minutes. Nevertheless, Matt elected to go ahead and start the ultramarathon, knowing from prior experience that pain can be unpredictable. Sure enough, he felt almost no discomfort in the knee during the race, and he was able to go the full 50 miles. The pain never returned.

Stories like this one are remarkably common, and they have a simple explanation: Movement is a drug. More precisely, physical exercise produces an analgesic effect similar to that of medications commonly used to treat pain. A 1984 study by Malvin Janal of the New

York State Psychiatric Institute found that a six-mile run stimulated an endorphin release in the brains of subjects that was equivalent to a 10 mg dose of morphine. Pretty cool. The comparison is overly simplistic, however, because in most respects, exercise is not at all like an injected or oral painkiller—it's much better.

Taking pain medication is like being given the answer to a math problem you're struggling with, whereas exercise is like figuring it out for yourself, which helps you not only in that particular test but in all future math tests. A dose of morphine will give you some relief from pain, but the relief won't last, and more importantly, it won't do anything to keep pain from negatively affecting your future training. Exercise, on the other hand, helps you navigate through your present pain experience in a way that empowers you to manage pain effectively for as long as you choose to continue challenging your body athletically.

The goal of this chapter is to set you up with a set of principles and methods that will enable you to self-manage pain with exercise. I will not be giving you a detailed step-by-step program that you can follow to manage pain of all types or even to manage any specific type of pain experience. That's not how Training as Treatment works. Remember, this method is more of an art than a science—a creative, experimental approach that, when done right, unfolds in unpredictable ways in each application. Even when I practice Training as Treatment with individual clients, I never know exactly where it will lead.

This doesn't mean I'm completely winging it. The principles and methods I'm about to describe establish the framework for a cohesive process that is certain to yield benefits if you practice it faithfully. But it does place some responsibility on you, requiring that you be open-minded and flexible, able to learn and adapt as you go. To be perfectly frank, if you want me or any other trainer to just tell you what to do, then Training as Treatment is not for you! As the case studies at the end of the chapter will make clear, your pain is unique and you are integral to the process, whether you work with a professional or go it alone.

Before I get down to the business of explaining this approach, let's first consider the mechanisms through which training treats pain. My intent in doing so is not to give you knowledge for knowledge's sake. Understanding the *why* behind the Training as Treatment approach will enable you to practice the method successfully.

HOW TRAINING TREATS PAIN

The acute pain reduction that often occurs during and after exercise is classified as *exercise-induced analgesia*. This effect is produced through a number of distinct mechanisms, which include the release of endogenous opioids (natural morphine), serotonin (natural Prozac), and endocannabinoids (natural cannabis) in the brain. Physiology aside, the very existence of exercise-induced analgesia is a reminder that pain is, in a very real sense, a choice that the organism makes in its own self-interest rather than something that is inflicted on it by forces outside its control. There is no stimulus that causes pain automatically; the organism always has a say in whether pain is experienced. From an evolutionary perspective, it's easy to understand why exercise-induced analgesia would aid survival. There are times when life depends on a creature's ability to run or fight or to act decisively in some other way, and pain cannot be allowed to stand in the way of such action.

Not only does a single bout of exercise reduce acute pain, but regular exercise layers on additional pain-mitigating effects. These effects are not thought to be related to observable healing in the affected tissue, improved flexibility, or any of the other factors that were once thought to contribute to pain reduction. This seems surprising until you're reminded that the relationship between pain and tissue damage is quite loose. But if exercise does not reduce pain in the expected ways, how does it? One mechanism is pain self-efficacy, as we will see in Chapter 8. Another is reduced pain sensitivity. Pain researchers sometimes use a pressure test to measure deep muscle tissue sensitivity in experimental subjects. A number of studies have shown that regular exercise reduces sensitivity to this type of pain, and it does so more reliably and effectively than nonexercise modalities, including pain education, massage, and stress management.

Not to be confused with reduced pain sensitivity is desensitization, which has more to do with fear of pain. As discussed previously, fear of pain provokes pain. In a typical case of nontraumatic musculoskeletal injury, fear might have little or no role in the initial onset of pain, but if pain persists in the absence of significant tissue damage, it is likely because a process of sensitization has occurred, whereby fear of activating the affected area has caused its use in performing certain movements to be experienced as painful. Counterintuitively, exercising this part of the body in the right way can reverse the sensitization process by violating the athlete's expectations—this is the "Wait, that was supposed to hurt" scenario, one example of which we saw in Chapter 3 with John Sherman.

Pain most often manifests when athletes push themselves more than they are accustomed to. An example of this type of "training error" is snowboarding for an entire morning after the first big snowfall of the winter, having not touched the board since the previous winter. Exercise mitigates this type of pain by elevating the threshold of what one is accustomed to so the tissues are less likely to be overwhelmed. Studies have shown, for example, that runners who are more accustomed to downhill running experience less pain after doing it than runners less accustomed to it.

There is a lot we still don't know about how exercise mitigates pain, and we may never have the full story. Nor does it matter, from a practical standpoint. Whereas pain scientists want to learn as much as they can about the underlying mechanisms for the sake of satisfying their curiosity and developing possible future care options, athletes just need to know how best to use exercise as a pain-management tool, so let's now talk about that.

HOW TO MANAGE PAIN WITH MOVEMENT

I'm not going to lie: When you're dealing with sport-associated pain, it is helpful to have someone like me to work with. It's not that any esoteric knowledge or advanced skill set is required to train through pain. One of the main points of *Pain and Performance* is that athletes are fully capable of managing pain effectively on their own. But I do have a ton of relevant experience, so when an athlete walks into Paragon Athletics and presents a particular pain situation, chances are I've seen something like it before and I have a good idea of where to start. I've got countless different exercises stored in my brain, and I'm able to conjure up new exercises as needed. And in most cases, I also know what might be an appropriate load type and dosage, and I can consider what other factors may be playing a role in someone's pain experience. I recognize that a lot of athletes might not have the same bandwidth or capacity to bring this level of problem-solving and creativity to a pain-management program. Still, you need not know everything I know to make real progress in self-managing pain, and you'll only get better as you gain experience in practicing Training as Treatment on yourself.

There are just two key principles you need to understand to get started with Training as Treatment: *exercise selection* and *progression*. Let's address both of them before looking at some specific examples of how I've applied these principles with real athletes.

EXERCISE SELECTION

There are countless different ways of exercising. Obviously, you need to have some criteria by which to narrow the options when your goal is to manage pain. The first of these is relevance. If you're a runner, for example, and pain in your right iliotibial band (or IT band, the large tendon running along the outer side of the thigh) is inhibiting your training, you'll want to do exercises that help you overcome this limiter. In this particular case, one of the exercises you'll want to do is running itself. Always train as close to normally as you can without experiencing a steady worsening of your pain or something that might qualify as a red flag. Doing so will prevent any unnecessary loss of sport-specific fitness, limit the anxiety and depression that come from not actively participating in your sport, serve as a gauge of progress, and even accelerate your return to full and unfettered training.

When you can't do your sport without exacerbating your pain experience, do something similar that doesn't make things worse. Let's say that your IT band pain (usually felt just above and outside the knee) is severe enough that it is inadvisable to do any amount of running. In this scenario, you might try bicycling or elliptical running as an alternative. This will keep you fit while giving the painful area time to calm down until you can ease back into running.

Strength training is almost always part of the solution to pain experiences, although it's not always clear exactly why strength training helps. What we do know is that appropriately selected strength exercises will guide your body back toward full functioning while also creating lasting changes that reduce the likelihood of a recurrence of the same issue. When I work one-on-one with athletes, I perform assessments that are designed to expose possible structural contributors to a given pain experience, such as a tendency for the pelvis to tip laterally during the stance phase of the running stride, which is commonly seen in runners with IT band pain. I know what you're thinking:

Isn't that exactly what physical therapists and trainers who are steeped in the structural model of athletic pain and injury do for the purpose of "correcting" incorrect movement patterns and structural imbalances?

Yes and no. It is true that certain strength exercises of the type a physical therapist or trainer might prescribe to "fix" a biomechanical or structural "problem" are effective in treating pain. However, they don't actually work by fixing movement patterns or structural imbalances. But again, it doesn't really matter why they work; it matters only that they are effective oftentimes. This is why I select strength exercises to address pain in much the same way I did when I myself was a structuralist, though I present them differently, without the verbiage that makes athletes feel fragile or defective. Your program should be fluid and flexible, responding to you and your needs. This is in contrast to the general prescription you might receive at a typical clinic.

One example of the type of exercise I might give an athlete with IT band pain is a side-lying plank. To do it, take off your shoes and lie on one side with a small weight or book balanced on the outside of the foot of the top leg. Begin with your bottom leg relaxed on the floor and your top foot positioned just behind the stationary foot and elevated a few inches off the floor. Now raise your top leg about 12 inches, swing it over the stationary leg, and lower it in front of the stationary foot of your bottom leg, all the while trying to keep the object from falling. Pause briefly with your foot a few inches off the floor, and then repeat the same movement (which you can think of as a parabola, or rainbow, movement) in reverse. Keep going back and forth at a slow, steady tempo for 3 minutes, pausing the clock to rest as necessary. Then flip over and repeat the exercise with the other leg.

A quick aside: You might wonder whether it is necessary to train both legs or arms or whatever if only one side is experiencing pain. The short answer is no. To the extent that your goal is to reduce pain in the affected area, it is sufficient to focus on that area. More often than not, however, I have my clients exercise both sides, because why not? Doing so reinforces the idea that despite your pain, you're still training, and pain reduction is not the only benefit of any strength exercise.

Another useful consideration in strength exercise selection is expectancy violation, where the idea is to move a part of your body that's giving you trouble in a way that defies the expectation of pain that often surrounds a pain experience. I find this approach helpful with certain types of pain experience, including hip tendinopathy. There's an exercise similar to the one I just described that I might have you do if you came to me with this issue. Take off your shoes and lie on the floor face up with one leg extended on the ground and the other raised straight up toward the ceiling while balancing a book on your foot. Because you're concentrating on the book, you're less likely to be thinking about your hip than you typically are when using it, and consequently, you will probably feel less pain. Experiences like this open the door to performing other hip movements with less pain or none at all.

Again, this is just an example. There's no single exercise I consider necessary for athletes with hip tendinopathy or any other sort of pain. Nor is any specific exercise helpful for every athlete with a given type of pain experience. Nor am I the only credible source of strength exercises helpful to athletes working to self-manage pain. I encourage you to explore other sources, such as Barbell Medicine, an online resource for strength coaching that caters to athletes seeking to train through setbacks.

The important thing to keep in mind is that there's no way to know ahead of time which specific exercises will benefit you most. All too many physical therapists work with printouts—exercise instruction sheets that they give to individual patients based on their injury type. They've got printouts for IT band friction syndrome, nonspecific low-back pain, swimmer's shoulder, and so on—a set exercise routine for every injury and every athlete who has that injury. It's a classic case of one size fits some. You wouldn't follow someone else's training plan when you're pain-free, would you? Then neither should you force yourself to adhere to a generic program when you do have pain.

Approach exercise selection with an experimental mindset. Choosing the wrong exercise—one that causes a bit too much pain or that you struggle with—is not a bad thing; it's part of an ongoing process of fine-tuning your training regimen to your body, which will change over time, ideally for the better (but not always). Embrace the art and be attentive to your body throughout the process, which should continue even after pain no longer limits your training. At this point, your fitness and performance goals become once again the primary criteria for your exercise selection, which doesn't necessarily mean you go back to training exactly the way you did before your pain experience. While we never wish them on ourselves, these episodes are opportunities to adjust our training and move a step closer to our personal optimal training formula. Too many athletes add useful variation to their training when dealing with pain and then fall back into a rut of doing the same things over and over. Maintaining enhanced variation in your exercise routine—indeed, making it less *routine*—will likely reduce the number and severity of pain experiences you face in the future.

I understand that as a regular athlete without formal schooling in strength and conditioning, you might not know where to begin with exercise selection—let alone how to keep the process going after you've returned to "normal" training. That's why I created the appendix of exercises at the back of this book and the additional resources available on the Paragon Athletics website. They're as close as you'll get to a printout from me!

Another factor to consider in selecting exercises is enjoyment— yes, enjoyment. After all, you chose to pursue your sport because you like it, so why shouldn't you also choose exercises you like when training through a pain experience? Not only is enjoyment intrinsically rewarding, but athletes also tend to be more consistent and disciplined in their training when they're having fun with it, which yields better results. For this reason, researchers, including Kathleen Sluka of the University of Iowa's Neuroscience Institute and Pain Research Program, advise clinicians to consider "patient preference" in designing exercise programs for pain management and injury rehabilitation.

PROGRESSION OF TRAINING THROUGH PAIN

Every athlete understands the principle of progression. You can't get fitter without making your training more challenging in one way or another. This is as true when you're training through pain as it is at any other time. But although the process is similar, the objective is different. When pain is not a major limiter, the goal of the training process is to increase fitness and performance. When pain is a significant limiter, the goal of training becomes removing this limiter and transitioning back to performance-focused training.

Think of the various methods you employ in your training as a tool kit. During pain experiences, one or more of the tools are temporarily removed from your tool kit. A cyclist with low-back pain, for example, might find that rides lasting longer than 90 minutes are intolerably uncomfortable. Hence the "tool" of longer rides may need to be removed from this athlete's tool kit for a period of time, and the goal of their strength training in this period becomes restoring the ability to comfortably ride longer than 90 minutes.

These two distinct training objectives—performance and the removal of limiters—are not mutually exclusive. You can and should continue to train for fitness and performance at the same time you're training to remove pain-related limiters. I recently met with a runner dealing with a painful hip abductor. "I guess I need to stop training for a while," he said to me in a tone of resignation that I've heard more times than I can remember. "Why?" I asked, then went on to explain to the runner that there was a lot of valuable work to be done in the meantime.

Strength training is something that all athletes (and nonathletes, frankly) should do not just when they are managing pain but all the time. Depending on their sport, I like to see athletes do a few full-body strength workouts each week plus daily complementary exercise sessions—miniworkouts focused on muscles and movements that tend to be neglected in an athlete's main sport. For an athlete who is already committed to this routine, the training process won't look much different in the midst of a pain experience than it will at any other time. Only the details will change, with certain exercises being added to address the issue and perhaps certain others being temporarily taken out of rotation pending improvement. There is no end point to the approach I teach. You just keep going, changing the specifics of your training based on where you are in the process.

With some (but not all) of the athletes I work with, the process actually begins with a step that doesn't involve getting sweaty: the step that I casually refer to as the "Pain Talk." Its purpose is to recontextualize the athlete's pain experience, giving them a conceptual foundation to make the most of the rest of the process (i.e., the part that does involve getting sweaty). In guiding an athlete toward a new perspective on pain, I explain that *pain* is not synonymous with *damage*, so they can be confident they aren't hurting themselves in a medical sense by performing exercises that induce a certain degree of pain. The goal, I suggest, is to be respectful but not fearful of pain as they progress through their training, neither seeking it out nor avoiding it.

The reason I don't initiate the Pain Talk right away with every athlete is that not every athlete is ready for it, and I can tell you from experience that going there prematurely can have disastrous consequences ("So you're saying it's all in my head?"). Therefore, I try my best to read each athlete and judge when, if ever, is the right time to educate them on pain. But even when I do get the timing right, this message does not take root immediately with every athlete. When it does, however, it makes a world of difference. Athletes are able to train with less anxiety and more confidence, which leads to greater consistency and faster improvement.

Obviously, your case is different. Instead of meeting with me one-on-one at Paragon Athletics, you're reading *Pain and Performance*. Ready or not, you've already received the Pain Talk! Jokes aside, the fact that you're still reading gives me confidence that you are in fact ready to see pain differently and to embrace the training method that's based on this view of pain. Am I right? Good. Now let's get sweaty.

Increase the Difficulty of Exercises

The logic of the training progression itself is simple: I present the athlete with exercises that are challenging but doable. When they've gotten the movements down, I advance them to fresh exercises that are challenging but doable at the level they've now reached, and so on. The various types of exercise I guide athletes through can be loosely grouped into three phases. An example of a phase 1 movement is the side-lying plank, which I referenced earlier as an exercise I might present to an athlete with IT band pain.

As this exercise becomes easier for the individual, I might replace it with the sliding wall squat, a phase 2 movement. Here's how to do it: Stand on your left foot near a wall on your right side. Press a folded towel against the wall with the outside of your right knee, first bending the knee 90 degrees so that the foot is extended behind you. Now lift your knee up as high as you can, keeping it pressed against the wall so that the towel slides along it. Next, reverse the motion, stopping when your right thigh is aligned with your left. Continue to raise and lower your knee for 3 minutes, resting as necessary. Then reverse your position and repeat the exercise with your left leg.

But wait—we're not done yet. As *this* exercise becomes easier for the athlete, I might swap it out for something like the forefoot Romanian deadlift, thereby advancing to phase 3. Stand on the ball of your right foot with a slight bend in the knee. Keeping the heel as high as possible, tilt forward at the hips and reach toward the floor with your right hand. Go as far as you can without increasing your knee bend or allowing your heel to drop, and then return to an upright position. Now reach toward the floor a second time and keep going for a cumulative 2 to 3 minutes, pausing your timer each time you lose your balance (which is likely!) or need to rest. To make the exercise even more challenging, do it while balancing on a two-by-four or holding a small weight in your reaching hand. Repeat the exercise on the opposite leg.

Incorporate a Variety of Exercises

In addition to increasing the difficulty level of your exercises as you make progress, it's beneficial to vary your exercises within each phase of the process. As I've mentioned, there's a large variety of strength exercises you can do for whatever part of your body might be troubling you, and it's best to do a variety of them instead of repeating the same ones over and over. A certain amount of repetition allows you to see progress, but this element of your training should be complemented with variation, where the challenge comes from novelty rather than from the inherent difficulty level of the movement. Keep in mind that the overarching objective of the process is not to get good at any specific set of exercises but to remove limiters on your ability to train.

As mentioned, the side-lying plank is an example of an exercise we might use in the first phase of the IT band pain protocol. Another hip strengthener that I might substitute for the side-lying plank at some point, for variation's sake, is the IT band wall squat. Stand with your left side facing a wall one large step away from it.

Lift and place your left foot against the wall about 18 inches above the floor, and shift your weight in the same direction, pressing the outside of the foot into the wall. While maintaining this pressure, squat down with your weight centered between your legs. (Note that you won't be able to do a very deep squat in this position.) Return to the starting position and then squat again, continuing for 3 minutes and pausing as necessary. Finally, reverse your position and repeat the exercise.

You might be wondering what determines whether a particular exercise is appropriate for phase 1, phase 2, or phase 3 of a progression. There are two main factors to consider: pain and the inherent difficulty of the exercise itself. When a particular part of the body is highly sensitive to pain, only a limited variety of strength exercises can be done comfortably. Also, independent of pain, some exercises are simply harder to do than others. In general, isometric exercises (where a muscle contraction is held for a period of time, as in most plank exercises) and isotonic exercises (where the amount of tension in the muscle is held constant while it contracts and relaxes, as in the IT band wall squat that was just described) are least painful for athletes dealing with highly pain-sensitive areas and are more doable for those who aren't especially strong or coordinated.

At the other extreme are ballistic or dynamic strength exercises— movements that involve jumping and other explosive actions. Examples are skipping rope, which is good for athletes working through Achilles tendon pain; backward box steps, which I use often as a phase 3 movement for athletes overcoming knee pain; kettlebell swings, which are a perfect fit for athletes seeing success in navigating through low-back pain; and rapid-tempo push-ups, which I've been known to give to athletes who've made a lot of progress in dealing with shoulder pain.

PACING YOUR PROGRESSION

The next question you might want to ask me is this: "How do you know when you're ready to transition to the next level of exercises?" Pain is the main indicator. When you get to the point where you're able to perform a given exercise with minimal pain, try stepping up to a more advanced phase 2 or 3 exercise. If that next exercise causes more pain than you're comfortable with, try something else. The one big qualifier I will add is that not all athletes experience pain the same way. The terms *persister* and *avoider* have been used to describe individuals who tend to push through pain and those who tend to shrink from pain, respectively. I don't love the terms because they carry a whiff of judgment, whereas in truth it's neither good nor bad to be a persister or an avoider. Furthermore, these terms imply that people are either one or the other, when in fact any single athlete might be a persister with certain pain experiences and an avoider with others.

Nevertheless, there is some usefulness in the underlying concepts of pain avoidance and pain persistence. Recognizing whether you lean in one direction or the other can help you decide how much pain to accept as you work through a progression like the one I've outlined. Pain avoidance is characterized by reflexive trepidation, hesitancy, or worry about using the affected body part. Pain persistence is revealed when athletes struggle to recognize that using the affected body part in a particular way isn't a good idea at the moment or struggle to alter their behavior in response to such recognition. The best results come when athletes find the Goldilocks zone between avoidance and persistence, where they recognize that they don't need to be afraid of moving or of the pain they may experience in doing so while also respecting their pain and not trying to withstand a degree of pain that is likely to slow their progress.

"How long will the entire process take?" you now ask. Again, the process has no end point, but it's natural to want to know how long it might take to get from the first phase to the point of returning to full performance-focused training. As the case studies presented in the next section show, when an athlete really commits to the process, they typically come out the other side in two to three months. But these examples all involve athletes who had been struggling with pain for a very long time before they came to me.

In cases of less persistent pain, athletes often return to full training within a few weeks and sometimes a few days. At the other extreme, a more stubborn pain experience may take many months to resolve even with full commitment to the process. In these cases, the athlete should be prepared for the possibility that some level of pain will always be with them. This doesn't mean the process or the athlete has failed or there's something wrong with them, nor does it necessarily mean the athlete can't fully enjoy their sport and achieve their goals with pain as a frequent companion. My advice is the same in all these cases: Try not to put a timeline on your recovery, trust the process, and avoid judging yourself.

AN INDIVIDUALIZED TRAINING AS TREATMENT PROCESS

Each and every pain experience is unique. This is why I work closely with each individual athlete to figure out a process that gets them back to full training. By this point in the chapter, I hope I've persuaded you that you can do the same with your pain experiences. Nevertheless, the following examples will help illustrate how different the process can look for each individual athlete. These case studies describe athletes who came to me in a state of real discouragement, not knowing the answer to their pain experience. The thing is, I didn't know the answer either! I knew only that the process I've just described would lead us to an answer, as I'm confident it will for you.

Case Study #1: Amber's Achilles

It had been over a year since Amber ran farther than 1 mile when she showed up at Paragon Athletics. She had been diagnosed with sural nerve entrapment, but I treated her simply as a runner with Achilles pain. In addition to ignoring her diagnosis, I dismissed the advice she'd been given to stop running and encouraged her to go ahead and run without fear of pain but also with respect for it. In the gym, Amber and I worked together to select strength exercises that involved the Achilles, but I saw Amber's active participation in the process as more important than the specific exercises.

With each new client, I try to get a feel for how useful it will be to converse openly about pain science. Amber seemed receptive to the initial bits of information I gave her, so I went ahead and taught her a lot about the biopsychosocial model, and it paid off. Within two months, her pain had receded to the point where she was able to log the same distances she was running before her troubles started.

Case Study #2: Victor's Knee

One of the more interesting clients I've ever had the pleasure of working with, Victor is a certifiable genius who teaches cosmology, or the study of the origins of the universe. Also a runner, Victor had been in physical therapy for knee pain for about five years—during which time his running had been severely limited and often interrupted—when he came to see me. X-rays and MRIs had yielded no diagnosis, which is just as well, because we know that diagnoses often do more harm than good.

Very seldom do I ask runners to modify their natural stride, but in Victor's case, I did so because I recognized that the ruminative nature that served him so well as a scientist might be less helpful with respect to his pain experience. Everyone focuses on their pain to some extent, but Victor *really* focused on his pain, so I put him on a treadmill and asked him to modify his footstrike slightly and hold small objects in his hands as he ran, for no other reason than to give him something else to pay attention to.

In the gym, we took a kitchen-sink approach to strength training. Victor wanted specific reasons for doing any given exercise, so I went further than I normally do in the direction of choosing "evidence-based" movements for him to perform. However, I was very careful to avoid presenting them to him with structuralist language that might exacerbate his sense of being weak or unbalanced or fragile. Within three months, Victor was pain-free. Neither he nor I will ever know what caused his knee pain or precisely what fixed it, and it doesn't matter.

Case Study #3: Meredith's Hip

An all-around outdoor enthusiast, Meredith was scheduled to have surgery to repair a labral tear and address what she'd been told was a femoroacetabular impingement (FAI) in her left hip. As is so often the case, the story Meredith had been told about her body by clinicians caused her to feel fragile, helpless, and fearful. In the beginning, the mere thought of using her hip was painful, so I focused her attention initially on the ankle of the same leg, which, in fact, was rather unstable. I gave her balance exercises and proprioceptive movements that drew her mind away from the hip.

The change in mindset that Meredith underwent over the next three months was stunning—in a good way. By the end of the process, she was actively seeking ways to provoke her remaining symptoms. Nothing is more painful to athletes with FAI than hip flexion (i.e., lifting the thigh), and when Meredith was ready, we introduced resisted hip flexion exercises, beginning with her pressing her knee against my hand and advancing from there. These exercises had the desired effect—which is to say they hurt—but Meredith no longer feared pain, and by embracing the process, she was able to do more and more with less and less pain and with ever greater confidence.

Case Study #4: Matt's Low Back

Most of my clients find me through word of mouth. Matt was an exception. A cyclist suffering from low-back pain that had kept him from riding consistently for two years and had severely impacted his quality of life, making it difficult for him to get out of bed some mornings and leading to depression, Matt was desperate enough, after two years of fruitless physical therapy, to search the Internet for athletic pain specialists, a process that brought him eventually to Paragon. I started him off with proprioceptive exercises, including the book-balancing exercise, just to get him comfortable "asking things" of his low back.

Because Matt was down in the dumps, I particularly focused on making things fun for him, having him do stuff like lie on his back and use the toe of his foot to trace lines I had drawn on the wall. At the same time, Matt had the mindset of a competitive athlete, so I repeatedly reinforced the idea that he was in training, not in therapy. He made rapid progress, graduating from one-on-one work with me to daily cycling on his own in about eight weeks.

Case Study #5: Maggie's Shoulder

I like Maggie's story because it demonstrates that training through a pain experience is largely a matter of building confidence—no different from training for competitive goals. Whether your goal is to improve your 10K run time or climb your first V5 boulder, your training must not only get you physically ready to do what you hope to do but also make you believe you can. It's very much the same in Training as Treatment, where the process is set up to prove to athletes through a step-by-step progression that they can do more with less pain, and that is exactly what it did for Maggie.

A nurse by vocation and a climber by avocation, Maggie had been in physical therapy for shoulder pain for two and a half years when

I met her. The experience had severely damaged her confidence. Maggie had been told her shoulder was hypermobile and dyskinetic, meaning she couldn't engage the musculature properly. She'd been taught to be so fearful of using the shoulder that she broke down in tears just talking about it during our initial consultation. I decided then and there to make confidence the number one priority of her training. To this end, I delivered the Pain Talk early on and continued to educate her about the biopsychosocial model thereafter so she could see for herself that some of the pronouncements that had been made about her body were baseless.

In my assessment, nothing could help Maggie more than getting back outside and reacquainting herself with the activities she loved and missed. We did some gym work together, but her first tentative test of the shoulder in the mountains went well, and after that, my role switched to that of coach. Maggie was experienced enough in her passions that her progression was mostly self-guided. My role was limited to providing regular electronic check-ins, where she told me how things were going and asked questions and I gave her encouragement and offered suggestions. At one point, I told her, "If you feel like you can do this on your own, you should." And I meant it. I measure my success by how quickly my clients decide they don't need me anymore, which in Maggie's case took just a few more weeks. As I often joke, Training as Treatment is a bad business model but a great care model.

CONDUCT YOUR OWN CASE STUDY

In reading the preceding case studies, you might find yourself thinking, "These are nothing more than sketches—Ryan's not giving me enough information to copy the things he did to help these athletes through their pain experiences," and you are right! Here's why: You can't manage your own pain successfully by repeating what someone else has done. What you can do is apply the process I've described in this chapter, the steps of which can be summarized as follows:

1. Recontextualize your pain through education on pain science.
2. Reflect on your persistence/avoidance tendencies with respect to pain.
3. Try various exercises that involve the painful area until you find ones that challenge it but not too much.
4. Continue to mix things up with your exercise selection for the purpose of challenging the painful area in different ways.
5. Progress incrementally from basic exercises, such as isometrics, that defy pain expectancies and desensitize the painful area toward more advanced exercises, such as ballistic movements, relying on reduced pain and improved strength or performance as cues that it's time to level up.

As you go, avoid looking too far ahead and making unfounded assumptions about what the next steps will look like or how quickly you'll get to them. This is easier when you've been through the process one or more times and seen that it got you where you wanted to go despite the lack of a turn-by-turn road map, after which you can truly trust in Training as Treatment. Until then, you'll need to take a leap of faith, believing that the method is at least worth trying and committing to see it through before passing judgment. In sharing the stories of Amber, Victor, Meredith, Matt, and Maggie, I hope to have inspired you to take that leap of faith and begin your own Training as Treatment journey.

8

OWN YOUR PAIN

In 1951, Harvard sociologist Talcott Parsons coined the term *sick role* to signify the identity and behaviors that patients are expected to adopt in societies such as ours where doctors possess great authority. It's something we all do to various degrees, mostly without realizing it. Even small things like the custom of addressing physicians as "Doctor So-and-So" are part of playing the sick role. Your doctor may call you Suzie or Dave, but don't you dare call your doctor Dave or Suzie!

I don't mean to imply that the sick role is nefarious. We all play roles of one kind or another in every relationship. There's a spouse role, a boss role, a student role—you get the idea. But roles are a bit like habits in that once adopted, they can be hard to break. In the medical arena, this is most likely to happen to patients with an illness or pain that is resistant to treatment. All too often, the care process continues for so long that the patient becomes psychologically dependent on it, such that treatment or therapy functions as a kind of substitute for healing or recovery.

I've mentioned previously that many of my clients come to Paragon Athletics as a last resort after they've hit a dead end in their efforts to find relief from their pain within the medical domain. Among these athletes are some who are clearly stuck in the sick role, having spent so much time in physical therapy that it has developed into an emotional crutch. Physical therapy is supposed to be a bridge from pain and dysfunction back to normal activity, but frequently it becomes an endless loop that's hard to break, and it's easy to see why—the entire experience undermines the patient's confidence in their ability to manage pain on their own.

Just ask Nick, a college wrestler turned motocross enthusiast who, at the time we met, had been in therapy for four years for low-back pain related to a fall he took on his dirt bike. Barely 30, Nick was so debilitated by his condition that he struggled to perform his duties as a mechanical engineer, and even his marriage began to suffer as a consequence of his distress. It wasn't long before I started to recognize signs of therapy dependence in Nick. He made frequent use of words like *fix*, which express a kind of passivity in the process, implying the expectation that any improvement in his condition would come about as the result of things I did rather than things he did. Another clue was Nick's then recent experience with postural restoration, an ultrastructuralist form of physical therapy (explained in Chapter 5) that seems almost as if it were designed to foster a patient's sense of fragility and dependence.

The clincher came when Nick divulged that his father also suffered from low-back pain. Research has shown that children of individuals with this condition are prone to develop it themselves, but the mode of transition isn't genetic—it's environmental. Among identical twins raised in different homes, low-back pain is more likely to emerge in those raised by a parent with low-back pain regardless of whether the parent is biological or adoptive.

Something about seeing a parent struggle with back pain creates a latent expectation of ending up in the same predicament. Having learned about Nick's family history, I knew I needed to kick him out of the nest, so to speak.

A good portion of the time I am with clients is spent in conversation, and this was true with Nick. We'd been working together for a few weeks when the moment seemed right to tell Nick the best next step in his process might be to find his own way using the tools he'd learned. I explained to him that I believed his real problem was not his back but therapy, or rather his relationship with it. I wouldn't usually lump my Training as Treatment approach together with things like postural restoration, but in this instance I did, since I felt that Nick needed to become independent of all types of clinicians to improve. Then again, a postural restoration therapist would never tell a patient, as I told Nick, "The best way I can help you is by getting out of the way." Indeed, my desire to make clients independent is perhaps the biggest difference between my method and others.

Nick's initial reaction to my little speech was one of surprise bordering on shock, but within minutes, his bewilderment began to give way to relief and acceptance. Nick's no dummy. He understood that he wasn't going to get better by doing more of the same. He'd come to me looking for something different, and that's precisely what I was offering him. We spent the remainder of the meeting hammering out some guidelines for the independent training Nick was to begin doing (a version of the Training as Treatment process described in Chapter 7)—a better solution, in his case, than depending on me for coaching or blowing up balloons to fix his back, as his postural restoration therapist was having him do.

It's no surprise that by following the guidelines I gave him, Nick made steady progress in both symptom management and function.

He's now back to riding dirt bikes, and he's able to work without limitations. Is he 100 percent pain-free? Of course not. But when I last checked in with him, Nick told me, "If I have a flare-up, I know how to handle it." That's exactly what I want to hear!

It's also pain self-efficacy in a nutshell. Defined by one researcher as "confidence regarding one's ability to function effectively while in pain," pain self-efficacy is arguably the main objective of Training as Treatment. An athlete who has confidence in their ability to train effectively despite pain and to manage pain effectively through training is an athlete who will be successful in these efforts. Sure, the method has other benefits—it keeps athletes from losing too much fitness when they are injured and makes the body more resilient against future injury—but its effect on pain self-efficacy has the greatest overall impact on the athletic experience. If you succeed in increasing your pain self-efficacy by practicing Training as Treatment, everything else will take care of itself.

Let's take a closer look at this all-important trait, how the medical system weakens it, and how to strengthen your belief in your ability to manage athletic pain effectively.

ADDRESSING LEARNED HELPLESSNESS

Every primer on self-efficacy begins with a reference to Albert Bandura, a Canadian-American psychologist who introduced the concept in 1977, defining *self-efficacy* (distinct from *pain* self-efficacy, defined above) as "a person's belief in their ability to succeed in a particular situation." Subsequent research by Bandura and others demonstrated that self-efficacy varies widely from person to person and that individuals with high levels of self-efficacy tend to be happier, healthier, and more successful. Studies also suggest that self-efficacy may be largely inherited (as much as 75 percent), but at the same time, it is highly responsive to experience.

Bandura believed that "mastery experiences," as he called them, are the most effective way to increase self-efficacy, and I tend to agree. Such experiences are almost always specific to a particular task, and the self-efficacy they engender is limited to that task, for the most part. If a boulderer has the mastery experience of solving a problem that was previously beyond their skill level, they are likely to gain a measure of self-efficacy that helps them complete even harder climbs in the future, but it won't necessarily make them think they can dunk a basketball or complete a backside quad 1980.

The concept of pain-specific self-efficacy originated with psychologist Jeffrey Dolce in 1986. In one study, Dolce and colleagues subjected 64 college students to a standard cold pressor test of pain tolerance, in which subjects immerse one hand in a bucket of ice water for as long as they can stand it. Prior to this test, the experimenters measured self-efficacy expectancies in the students, or how long they thought they could last before withdrawing their hand from the bucket. It turned out that expectancies strongly predicted actual pain tolerance, influencing subjects' immersion times to a greater degree than offering monetary incentives or setting quotas.

In the 1990s, Michael Nicholas of the University of Sydney's Pain Management Research Institute took these ideas further, demonstrating that pain self-efficacy and physical functioning could be increased through a cognitive behavioral pain-management program. In 2007, Nicholas created a standardized questionnaire that has since been used to assess and measure changes in pain self-efficacy. This questionnaire is presented in Figure 8.1.

Figure 8.1 Pain Self-Efficacy Questionnaire

Rate how confident you are that you can do the following things at present, despite the pain. A score of 0 indicates "not at all confident" and 6 indicates "completely confident."

	0	1	2	3	4	5	6
I can enjoy most things, despite the pain.							
I can do most of the household chores (e.g., tidying up, washing dishes), despite the pain.							
I can socialize with my friends and family members as much as I used to, despite the pain.							
I can cope with my pain in most situations.							
I can do some form of work, despite the pain. ("Work" includes housework, paid work, and unpaid work.)							
I can still do many of the things I enjoy doing, such as hobbies or leisure activities, despite the pain.							
I can cope with my pain without medication.							
I can still accomplish most of my goals in life, despite the pain.							
I can live a normal lifestyle, despite the pain.							
I can gradually become more active, despite the pain.							

Unfortunately, at the same time Nicholas and others were developing and testing nonmedical means of increasing pain self-efficacy, the medical establishment was working toward ensuring that virtually all pain was treated pharmaceutically. Medical historians trace the origin of this monopolization to the advent of the gate control theory of pain described in Chapter 6. This theory shifted how scientists and doctors thought about pain in ways that made it possible to see pain as a problem in itself, distinct from any particular cause. In turn, this shift in thinking led to the emergence of multidisciplinary pain clinics and pain-focused treatment centers. Next came a raft of professional pain associations intended to advance the interests of clinicians and researchers focused on pain treatment.

And then came the opioid epidemic.

Obviously, it's not quite that simple. But even some doctors and researchers now admit that this mother of all unintended consequences, which has claimed more than 400,000 lives worldwide, was an almost inevitable result of the medicalization of pain. In a candid personal essay published by the Kaiser Permanente Washington Research Institute, physician Eric Larson, who studies resilience in older populations, wrote,

> Doctors and patients alike were led to believe that drugs like Oxycontin, Vicodin, and Percocet were the magic solution to one of life's universal problems. Our field made a conscious effort to "medicalize" pain as though pain alone were a disease state. Pain became a new vital sign, so we adopted the idea that health care teams should routinely monitor pain. Many believed it was the provider's job to not just reduce pain, but to eradicate it. At the same time, we were falsely taught we could easily do this with prescription opioids, which were thought to be effective, nonaddictive, and mostly safe.

The warlike death toll only hints at the overall cost of the opioid epidemic. For every person who's lost their life to an overdose, there are many more whose lives have been irreversibly ruined by addiction. Lesser consequences of this man-made catastrophe extend into the sports arena, where countless athletes have been prescribed painkillers for pain experiences they could have worked through without medication. But the harm done to athletes by the medicalization of pain goes beyond opioids and even beyond messaging like that insidiously self-efficacy-robbing advertising tagline cited at the very beginning of this book: "When pain says you can't, Advil says you can." If you've ever been told by a clinician that you're prone to injury because of an imbalance in your body, you've been negatively affected by the medicalization of pain. If you've ever gotten platelet-rich plasma therapy or cold laser treatment for an injury, you've been negatively affected by the medicalization of pain. If you've ever been led to believe that you needed a clear diagnosis to get past pain, you've been negatively affected by the medicalization of pain. And so on.

Not oblivious to this state of affairs, some clinicians and scientists within the sports medicine establishment have begun to sound the alarm. In 2019, for example, Daniel Friedman of Monash University and Karim Khan of the University of British Columbia penned an educational review titled "Preventing Overdiagnosis and the Harms of Too Much Sport and Exercise Medicine" for the *British Medical Journal*. In it, they describe the emergence of an institutional structure that empowers sports medicine clinicians to turn athletes into patients the moment they experience any pain beyond the norm. The four key elements of this system, according to Friedman and Khan, are (1) the belief among clinicians that more intervention yields better outcomes; (2) so-called diagnosis creep, whereby the definition of injury keeps expanding; (3) the commercialization of sports medicine and injury treatment (i.e., sports pain treatment as cash cow);

and (4) the increased accessibility of sports medicine and injury treatment services.

I would add a fifth element: how athletes think about pain. There was a time, not that long ago, when athletes learned how to think about pain from coaches. If your knee began to bother you at soccer practice, you would tell your coach, who might make some sensible adjustments to your training and play. But nowadays, if your knee begins to bother you at soccer practice, it is likely that you will bypass your coach and tell a doctor, whose advice is likely to be something along the lines of "You have patellar tracking disorder and ought to consider lateral release surgery to correct the subluxation that currently makes you prone to injury."

Don't let the glibness of this illustration mislead you. The modern notion that athletes are helpless in the face of pain and must depend on medical professionals to deal with pain experiences is so pervasive that even some of our greatest athletes parrot the language of sports medicine clinicians. Recently, I listened to an interview with John Gill, who is regarded as the godfather of the sport of bouldering. Born in 1937, Gill preceded John Sherman and inspired "Verm" (as he is affectionately known) in much the same way Verm inspired me. Anyway, toward the end of the interview, Gill was asked if he had any advice for the people listening.

"I would counsel people these days not to get into bouldering, as a matter of fact," he said, "because of all the spinal damage it did to me."

I couldn't believe my ears. Gill was 84 years old when he spoke these words, and he'd just finished telling the interviewer that he was still capable of performing a front lever that any strong climber would envy and about which he'd said, "I still get a feeling of lightness doing these and other exercises." Yet despite his impressive level of fitness and his continuing enjoyment of testing his body, Gill thought of himself as a broken-down old man and warned others against ending up like him—able to perform a lever at 84 years old, albeit with some pain—as if sedentary persons of the same age don't have pain!

I'm not pinning blame on John Gill, who is more of a victim in this scenario. But his words illustrate just how much personal autonomy athletes have lost to the sports medicine establishment. In cautioning would-be boulderers to "Do as I say, not as I do," this legendary athlete was essentially doing the doctors' work for them not only by discouraging pain self-efficacy but also by encouraging something that goes hand in hand with it: kinesiophobia.

OVERCOMING THE FEAR OF MOVEMENT

Humans are hardwired to avoid pain and painful stimuli. In order for this instinct to work effectively, we must be capable of learning from painful experiences. Such learning is mediated partly through fear. When something we do results in pain, we are likely to fear that thing in the future, and this fear keeps us from repeating the painful experience.

For athletes, this mechanism can become problematic when pain is experienced during training and competition. A cyclist who feels knee pain while riding could begin to fear the activity and might even continue to fear it after it's no longer painful, a conditioning effect that, although natural, doesn't serve the interests of the cyclist. The term for this type of fear of movement is *kinesiophobia*, and it is most pronounced in those who suffer from chronic pain or are returning from a major injury. Fearing movement is not always a bad thing—we want to be wary of movements that are truly harmful—but this emotion becomes maladaptive in athletes who fear specific movements more than is necessary to protect themselves from harm. In these cases, kinesiophobia becomes a self-fulfilling expectation, causing athletes to experience more pain and regain function more slowly than athletes whose fear of pain hasn't taken on a life of its own.

Kinesiophobia has been widely studied in athletes returning to sport after anterior cruciate ligament (ACL) repair. In one study led by Mark Paterno of Cincinnati Children's Hospital, 40 athletes were tracked for two years after undergoing reconstructive knee surgery. Those who exhibited the highest levels of kinesiophobia were found to be less active, perform less well in a single-leg hop test, and have a higher likelihood of reinjuring the affected knee. Sometimes, the thing we fear is the problem. Other times, fear itself is the problem. When athletes fear movement, more often than not, fear is the problem.

This fear is actively stoked by the sports medicine establishment. I'm not suggesting that doctors and physical therapists huddle together in darkened rooms, plotting to exacerbate athletes' fear of exercising. However, the notion that exercise is dangerous follows naturally from the core axioms of the structural model of athletic pain and injury, according to which pain always signals injury and injury is always the result of flawed movement patterns rooted in musculoskeletal imbalances.

Consider that old, familiar legal disclaimer: "Consult your physician before starting an exercise program." This might be the craziest eight-word sentence in the history of language. Exercise is unequivocally healthy for almost everyone, something that—with rare exceptions—every living person should do. It makes absolutely no sense at all for doctors to be gatekeepers to physical activity. Imagine being told to consult your physician before adding more fresh vegetables to your diet, or starting a meditation practice, or falling in love, or adopting a kitten, or doing anything else that is good for you. I have no doubt you'd laugh in the face of anyone who had the temerity to utter something so absurd, yet no one bats an eye when told to seek a doctor's permission to ride a bicycle. True, few people actually heed this caution, but this doesn't mean the sports medicine establishment hasn't succeeded in convincing most people, including most athletes, that exercise can be dangerous. After all, what's the first thing most athletes do when a new pain experience limits their training? They call a doctor!

BUILDING PAIN SELF-EFFICACY

Let me be clear: There is no need to call a doctor every time you experience pain in the course of doing your sport. Instead, call on your own ability to manage pain, possibly with the help of a coach or trainer. In doing so, you will avoid the many negative consequences associated with going down this path and take a step toward pain self-efficacy and away from kinesiophobia. You might not be as dependent on medical pain "fixers" as Nick and some of the more desperate athletes who come to me for help, but even if that is the case, you're probably not as self-reliant as you could be. My goal is to get you to the point where you own your pain, by which I mean you don't cede control of pain management to a doctor, physical therapist, or anyone else and also that you don't let pain control you. Owning your pain doesn't necessarily mean steadfastly refusing to seek help from clinicians. But it does mean that you do so selectively and that you never let it lead to a relationship of dependency.

One of the surprising things I discovered when the COVID-19 pandemic forced me to shift to video appointments with most of my clients was that being separated from them actually facilitated the process of cultivating self-reliance. Athletes simply can't be as dependent on me at a distance, which is a good thing. Like any form of self-efficacy, pain self-efficacy can't be pulled out of thin air but requires experiential proof. In much the same way you can't go out and run a three-hour marathon unless you've proven to yourself that this goal is within reach through the training process, you can't manage athletic pain with confidence until you've experienced a success or two in training through pain. In my role as a trainer, the most I can do is coax athletes to a place where they are willing to embrace the process with some expectation of success.

TAKE ADVANTAGE OF YOUR FREEDOM

The approach I use to guide athletes toward embracing Training as Treatment is informed by an experience I had back on the horse farm in Hot Springs, Arkansas, when I was a boy. My dad and I were leading a pair of thoroughbreds from the paddock to the barn when the horse I was responsible for reared up. My reflexive response was to pull back on the bit shank, which nearly caused the animal to flip over like a motorcycle executing a wheelie gone wrong. Afterward, my dad explained with his usual sangfroid that the next time a horse reared while I was leading it, I should do the exact opposite of what I had done, giving it more slack.

"Horses don't want to flip," he said. "If you give them the freedom to avoid it, they won't. Take away that freedom, and they just might."

People are the same way, I've discovered. The worst thing I could do in the effort to instill pain self-efficacy in an athlete is to come on strong with my biopsychosocial shtick. Embracing the Training as Treatment method as a path to successful pain management has to feel like the athlete's own idea. So instead of lecturing my clients about how everything they've been told about pain and injury is wrong, I use motivational interviewing and other communication techniques (as discussed in Chapter 5) to bring them along to a place of open-minded receptiveness.

Admittedly, effective motivational interviewing requires real-time verbal interaction between interviewer and interviewee. But I'm a clever guy (and also resourceful), and I've come up with what I consider to be a very close approximation of the process I go through with my clients in a format that you can use on your own right now—or any time. What follows is a sequence of questions and statements similar to those you would hear from me in the context of a one-on-one appointment. Answer them in any way you please, either by speaking your answers aloud, saying them in your thoughts, typing them out, or writing them down freehand in the style of journaling. This exercise has the most value if you have a current pain experience. If you don't, you can either answer from the perspective of your most recent pain experience or wait for your next one (and there will be a next one).

PAIN SELF-EFFICACY
MOTIVATIONAL INTERVIEW

Do you experience pain when performing one or more sports-related activities?

Do you believe that the painful area is damaged?

Here's an interesting fact for you to consider as you mull over these questions: research shows that most athletes experiencing pain not resulting from a traumatic injury have little or no underlying tissue damage, and even when they do, the damage is not the actual cause of the pain in any simple sense.

Are you open to the possibility that the pain you're experiencing is not caused by significant tissue damage?

Are you fearful that continuing to train might make your pain worse?

Here's an interesting fact for you to consider as you mull over these questions: research shows that exercise—strength training in particular—tends to reduce pain and improve function more often than it has the opposite effect.

Are you open to the possibility that training in a sensible way will help you get past your current pain experience?

Here's an interesting fact for you to consider as you mull over these questions: according to research, individuals who have a high degree of fear of movement-related pain take longer to return to full function than those who fear movement less.

Are you open to the possibility that addressing your fear of movement will help you return to full functioning quicker?

Do you fear pain itself, independent of any damage it might signal?

Here's an interesting fact for you to consider as you mull over these questions: studies suggest that inducing tolerable amounts of pain in a progressive manner through exercise is the most effective way to lessen this fear.

Are you open to the possibility that seeking out a certain amount of pain instead of trying to avoid all pain might be the best way to stop your fear of pain from limiting your training?

How confident are you in your ability to manage pain on your own?

Here's an interesting fact for you to consider as you mull over these questions: research indicates that people who have confidence in their ability to manage their own pain are usually right and that people who lack such confidence can acquire it.

Are you open to the possibility that you can gain confidence in your ability to manage your pain on your own?

As you can see, there are a few choice scientific facts sprinkled among the questions, which is not the usual thing in motivational interviewing but a calculated move on my part. As important as personal experience is in developing pain self-efficacy and overcoming kinesiophobia, beliefs are also important. You are far more likely to have success in using the Training as Treatment approach to owning your pain if you buy into it conceptually right from the start. It is for a similar reason that pain science education is now commonly used in the treatment of chronic pain, and studies show it works. In 2020, the journal *Physical Therapy Rehabilitation Science* published a review of past research on the effects of pain science education on kinesiophobia and pain severity in patients with chronic pain. A total of eight studies involving 369 patients were analyzed by the authors, who concluded that pain science education has "a positive effect on the improvement of pain and kinesiophobia in patients with chronic pain."

HOW TO MANAGE PAIN WITH EXERCISE

Among the most important objectives of this book is that of persuading you that you can successfully self-manage athletic pain through exercise. Naturally, you'll have to actually see it work before your pain self-efficacy can be fully maximized, which, like it or not, can't happen until you develop a new pain episode that requires you to modify your training. When you do, you'll be in a better position to train through your pain and get the "mastery experience" you need to tackle the next pain episode with greater confidence if you're already following a good strength program. In that case, all you have to do is modify your training in the manner laid out in Chapter 6. The stages of building pain self-efficacy are summarized below.

PROCESS FOR BUILDING
PAIN SELF-EFFICACY

Stage 1:   Start a strength training routine if you don't have one already.

Stage 2:   Continue training and doing your strength routine until you develop a pain experience that affects your main sport.

Stage 3:   Adjust your activity in your primary sport so that your pain remains at a tolerable level and doesn't get worse over time.

Stage 4:   Temporarily suspend any strength exercises in your normal routine that cause a level of pain that feels excessive. Introduce one or more exercises that involve the painful area and don't cause excessive pain.

Stage 5:   When the new strength exercises become easy and/or when your pain level decreases noticeably, replace one or more of these exercises with others involving the painful area that are more challenging and/or stimulate a little more pain. When these exercises in turn become easy and/or your pain level decreases further, swap them out once more. While the specifics depend on the location, nature, and severity of your pain, in most instances, this process starts off with isometric exercises, where you hold a muscle contraction, and terminates with explosive movements.

Stage 6:   At the same time you're going through the process detailed in stage 5, gradually reintroduce elements of your normal training in your primary sport as your pain allows.

Let's look at a specific example of the six-step process I've just outlined. Suppose you develop pain in your right shoulder. If you were to seek a diagnosis for it—which would be a mistake—you might be told you have medial epicondylitis, but what you really have is shoulder pain. If you're a tennis player, you might have to modify your game for a while, perhaps avoiding overhead swings. If you're a swimmer, you might have to soften your pull or switch to breast-stroke for the time being.

In the gym, you'll want to start the symptom modification process with one or more exercises that use the painful shoulder in a way that distracts your attention from it and perhaps also with one or more exercises that create a sense of safety by imposing a gentle, consistent load. One possibility is the teacup exercise. Fill a cup with water and balance it on the palm of your right hand with your arm raised overhead. Now rotate your palm clockwise as far as you can, trying not to spill. When you reach the limit of your range of motion, begin to rotate your shoulder forward, which will cause you to simul-taneously lower your hand and raise your elbow, allowing your hand to continue spinning. From this position, you will be able to once again rotate your wrist. Do so while lowering your arm, causing the cup to pass under your bicep along the way. Complete the motion by now raising your arm as you rotate at the shoulder, elbow, and wrist until you end up back in the position you started in. By concentrat-ing on the complex coordination of this movement pattern and on avoiding spillage, you will distract your attention from your shoulder and give your shoulder a better workout than you might be able to do with a more traditional exercise.

Once you've mastered the teacup drill and other phase 1 move-ments, introduce greater challenges such as isometric strength exer-cises. For the shoulder, an isometric exercise can be as simple as pressing your right palm into a wall as forcefully as you can with your elbow bent 90 degrees. Keep pressing continuously until you reach either the point of fatigue or the limit of your pain tolerance, whichever comes first. When you're ready for phase 3, try ballistic movements such as bouncing a stability ball against a wall, which is far more taxing than you'd think. This is also a great time to begin reintroducing any remaining sport-specific movements you previously put on pause.

In offering these examples, I don't want to give the impression that the process is identical for every athlete with similar symptoms. Remember, a major objective of the process is developing confidence in your own ability to navigate your way through a pain experience. You'll be more successful in this effort if you experiment, pay close attention to how your body responds to the things you try, and continually adapt based on what you notice. The recipe is different for each athlete, and because you alone can feel your body, you are in a better position than anyone to figure out the right recipe for moving through a given pain experience. There's also an element of unpredictability in every case, making it impossible to apply a cookie-cutter approach effectively. For example, in working through a recent pain episode in my left shoulder, I discovered that it responded surprisingly well to heavier loads, so I went ahead and applied them even though this was not what I or anyone else would consider the textbook approach to managing the early stages of a situation like mine.

I understand that many athletes feel daunted by the prospect of having to figure things out for themselves where pain is concerned, which is itself a sign of low pain self-efficacy. This is why I have created the example training programs you'll find in the Appendix and at paragonathletics.com. It's not unfair to think of these exercise sequences as the default programs I would administer to athletes if for some reason I were not permitted to communicate with them or gather any information that might be used to adjust their programs as they go. Having access to these programs will spare you the trouble of having to discover or come up with exercises on your own. I urge you to remain as open as possible to adapting the program as you go.

PAIN AND PROGRESS

There are a few key things to keep in mind throughout the process, especially if you're starting off with either a very low level of pain self-efficacy (indicated by anxiety and doubt about the process and perhaps also by the urge to consult a physician or physical therapist) or a very high level of kinesiophobia (which almost always manifests as a palpable fear of performing exercises that might induce pain). The most important things to keep in mind are that any pain you experience is not evidence of a medical problem and you are not hurting yourself by going through the six-step process outlined earlier in this chapter. Another thing to keep in mind is that your progress is unlikely to be linear. If you experience a flare-up in your pain at some point, don't take it as an indication that you've done something wrong. It's actually an indication that you're doing things right. Getting through the process without any setbacks usually means you went about it too conservatively. Don't forget, Training as Treatment is a method of pain management, not a method of pain avoidance. Inducing a certain amount of discomfort is the goal, not an unfortunate side effect of pursuing some other goal.

There is such a thing as being too aggressive, naturally. As I've said previously, if your pain intensifies over time, you're doing too much. Even in this scenario, though, there's nothing to be alarmed about. To draw an analogy, if you pick a level 5 marathon training plan when you ought to have picked a level 3 plan, and four weeks into it, you find yourself feeling more and more fatigued every time you run, you don't call your physician and say, "Doc, I think I'm sick!" What you do instead is call on your common sense and dial your training back to the level 3 plan you should have gone with in the first place. Treat a pattern of worsening pain the same way. Successfully improvising your way through a setback in your pain-management process will give your pain self-efficacy a big boost. One doesn't go seeking flare-ups, of course, but they are excellent opportunities to take a step forward in owning your pain.

RED FLAGS THAT MERIT MEDICAL INTERVENTION

Don't delete your doctor's contact information just yet. There are a few rare events that, should they occur during exercise, truly are cause for seeking medical help. These universally recognized red flags are as follows:

numbness or weakness,

incontinence,

significant bruising or swelling,

deformation (e.g., a bulge in your lower abdomen),

seizure,

loss of consciousness,

confusion,

or a gut feeling that something's not right.

Contrary to what has been said about me by certain detractors, who like to paint me as a fire-breathing radical who loves pain, I'm actually quite reasonable. I will be the first to admit that if in the middle of a workout you suddenly poop your pants and lose all feeling in your right leg before passing out, you should see a doctor ASAP.

9

Everything Matters

My friend Joe, who shares my passion for climbing, has come to me a number of times over the years for help in dealing with various pain experiences, most but not all of them related to bouldering. His most recent setback was a pesky elbow issue that had Joe feeling both concerned and baffled. It started after a camping trip during which he'd used an axe to split a log—just one—for use in a campfire. Weeks later, to his growing dismay, the elbow still hurt.

"I don't understand how something so small could mess me up like this," he said.

Knowing Joe as I do, I felt pretty sure chopping wood was not the singular cause of his pain. To test my hunch, I changed the subject, asking Joe a series of questions about how things were going for him. Next thing I knew, my friend was in tears, having opened up about the financial strain that COVID-19 had placed on the climbing gym he owned in Phoenix, his fear that this new injury would put an end to his bouldering, and his anxiety about aging. I took the opportunity to explain to him the concept of allostatic load, or the sum total of different types of stress a person is under, which has a proven connection to pain. Specifically, when allostatic loads are high—whether it's because of work stress, relationship stress, or any other kind of stress—new pain experiences are more likely to occur and existing pains are prone to intensify.

When I present these ideas to new clients—many of whom I don't know as well as I know Joe—I usually get one of two reactions. Some scoff at the notion that what they regard as a purely psychological stimulus (stress) could have a purely physical effect (pain). A few even take offense, misconstruing my message as an insinuation that their pain is "all in their head." We can all accept the fact that our psychology plays a role in our performance, but to acknowledge that it plays a role in our pain experience is, for many of us, a much tougher pill to swallow. This phenomenon is known as a *stereotype threat*, which is defined as a fear of being "labeled" on the basis of one's behavior—or in this specific case, a fear of being labeled weak or crazy due to experiencing pain that has no physical cause. On the other end of the spectrum, plenty of my clients readily accept the stress-pain connection, often with no small measure of relief, understanding that it gives us more ways to address their pain than if the cause were purely physical. Joe, I'm happy to say, fell into the second camp and was all the more accepting when I assured him that we would still use exercise as one tool to bring his elbow around.

Pain is not unique in being neither wholly physical nor entirely psychological. *Nothing* in human experience is ever purely physical or purely psychological. We speak of physical and psychological causes and effects as if these things were completely distinct, when in fact they are far from it. Pain is always both physical and psychological, and unless you were raised by wolves and now live alone on an isolated island, it's always social as well. This is the true meaning of the biopsychosocial model of pain. Many who claim to understand the model think of pain as being something like a dinner plate with three separate items on it—biological, psychological, and social—when in reality, pain is more like a soup where these three key ingredients are all mixed together. And that's a good thing, as it allows clinicians like me, whose job is to help people manage pain, to work on all three dimensions of pain with any single technique. My primary tool happens to be exercise, which is commonly regarded as physical, but as we've seen, it carries psychological benefits. There are also social benefits to exercise. Consider how important athletics are to your social identity. Training through pain instead of trying to heal through passive rest enables "injured" athletes to maintain their sense of identity.

Stress is also three-dimensional. For convenience, individual stressors can be classified as physical (lack of sleep), psychological (financial worries), or social (marriage trouble), but all stressors end up in the same soup. But the similarities between pain and stress go even deeper—so deep that some scientists regard them as almost the same thing. What is certain, in any case, is that stress of all kinds contributes to pain, and stress management, therefore, is an important part of pain management.

THE STRESS-PAIN CONNECTION

The term *allostasis* refers to the ability of an organism to absorb and adapt to pain and stress. Allostatic load, then, is the cumulative burden placed on this ability by the various stressors an organism is exposed to. Although stress has negative connotations, it is not inherently unhealthy. On the contrary, many of the ways our bodies and minds adapt to stress make us healthier and stronger. Exercise is a great example. Physical exercise is a stressor, but we can apply it in a controlled way that makes us fitter.

Only when too much of the wrong kinds of stress pile up does stress become harmful. Too much exercise is known to cause injury (and I'm talking about real injuries, such as stress fractures), burnout, and overtraining syndrome, a form of chronic fatigue affecting high-level athletes who push themselves too hard. Certain physical stressors, such as toxic chemicals, are unhealthy even in small amounts. But many of these stressors also provoke healthy adaptive responses when exposure doesn't exceed a critical threshold. The scientific term for this effect is *hormesis,* and it is similar to the mechanism employed by many vaccines, where intentionally exposing the body to a bit of a virus protects it against subsequent natural exposure to a lot of a virus. At the other extreme, some psychological stressors, including the stress of a demanding job that a person loves passionately, can be tolerated in very large amounts and become harmful only in extreme amounts.

Among psychological stressors, control plays a crucial role in determining whether a particular stressor functions as eustress (good stress) or distress (bad stress). In general, people tolerate stressors they choose (such as a challenging job) better than stressors that choose them (like financial hardship). The less control you feel in a stressful situation, the more likely it is to negatively impact your physical and mental health.

Pain itself is a stressor, and all the more so when it seems to be beyond your control, as it so often does. But the causal link between pain and stress operates in both directions. In other words, not only does persistent pain induce a stress response, but persistent stress of other types appears to trigger, or at least exacerbate and prolong, pain in some individuals. The word *persistent* is key here. Acute, or short-term, stress is known to increase pain tolerance. This is why we tend to experience more pain after the fight is over than during the fight. But in stressful situations that are long-lasting, like being bullied at school or harassed in the workplace, pain sensitivity tends to increase while pain tolerance declines.

This is easy to understand on an intuitive level. If you've ever gone through a particularly stressful period of your life, you know that it places you in a frazzled state where even the smallest setback—such as a minor pain experience—provokes an exaggerated emotional response. When your capacity to deal with stress is exceeded, sensations that might not normally register as pain become painful, and common pain experiences can seem unbearable.

The stress-pain relationship varies significantly among individuals based on genetic, physiological, and behavioral factors. For example, people with high levels of trait anxiety—meaning they are generally prone to feeling anxious—exhibit heightened reactivity to situational stress. Research has shown that these same individuals also exhibit higher pain sensitivity and lower pain tolerance compared to people with low trait anxiety, which is unsurprising in light of the strong link between stress and pain.

Anxiety has both genetic and environmental underpinnings. If you had an anxious parent, you're more likely to share the same predisposition. But you are also likely to tend toward anxiety if you were raised by an adoptive parent who had no genetic relationship to you but had an anxious personality. Environmental influences can affect how you experience pain in other ways as well. Another example of this is facing adverse life experiences in childhood. Interestingly, individuals who experience either very high levels of psychological trauma or very few adverse life experiences while growing up tend to be more sensitive to and less tolerant of pain as adults than individuals who experienced moderate levels of psychological trauma in childhood.

The upshot of all this science is that in every living human there exists the potential for stress to manifest as pain. And in athletes, there is the extra potential for stress to manifest as pain related to training. But this potential is not equal in all athletes. In some, due to a combination of biological, psychological, and social influences, stress may quickly and frequently translate into pain, whereas in others, only the highest allostatic loads (which may include high training loads) will manifest this way.

Stress can produce pain in even the toughest athletes. I helped ultrarunner Helen Galerakis prepare for a 2019 attempt to break the

FKT (Fastest Known Time) for traversing the Arizona Trail, which extends 800 miles from the northern border to the southern border of the state. To succeed, she would have to cover more than 50 miles of unforgiving terrain a day for more than two weeks. And if that wasn't pressure enough, Helen's attempt got a lot of media hype, so if she failed, she would do so publicly.

Feeling the pressure, she slept poorly the night before she started. The following night, around 3 a.m., I received an urgent text message from Helen, who was then at the bottom of the Grand Canyon. Evidently, the long, steep descent into the canyon had done a number on her right knee, and she was in pain. Worried that she now faced a choice between continuing at the cost of destroying her knee and quitting at the cost of wasting a year's preparation, she asked me to come out and examine her ASAP.

I met Helen and her crew at the south rim of the canyon the next day. Her leg was visibly swollen just above and outside the knee, indicating inflammation of the IT band, and she moved in a stiff-legged fashion that *looked* painful. Despite these clear indications that Helen's pain had a physical cause, I knew that stress—her lack of sleep, the high stakes of her undertaking, the spotlight she was under—was also a contributing factor. Had there been less at stake, I would have advised her to take a few days off to let the knee calm down, but instead I told her I believed she could safely continue. Was I 100 percent certain of this? No. But I was hopeful that hearing this assurance would lighten Helen's allostatic load just enough to enable her to achieve her goal.

I saw Helen again four days later and 275 miles farther south in Globe, Arizona. Amazingly, her pain and swelling were gone, and her stride was as smooth as butter. Think about that for a second: Hard running combined with other stressors had caused Helen to experience severe pain in a critical joint. Then additional hard running combined with a reduction of other stressors had eliminated her pain. It's an incredible example of the extent to which "non-physical" stressors can influence athletic pain, for better or worse.

To be clear, I'm not suggesting that Helen (who did achieve her goal despite the delay caused by her knee situation) somehow brought her pain on herself unnecessarily by allowing herself to become stressed out. What's true for her is true for millions of athletes, and it's no character flaw. But there's a reason I feel compelled to make this point clear. Unfortunately, there exists in our society a deeply entrenched double standard around biological and psychosocial contributors to pain that makes it difficult for professionals to address the latter with clients. If I told you the knee pain you're experiencing when you ride your bike is caused by your kneecap's failure to track properly, in essence blaming your pain experience on your body, you probably wouldn't feel insulted. But if I told you that I believe the high level of life stress you're currently experiencing is probably contributing to your knee pain, you might take it personally. I know this because I deal with it all the time. When I say, "I think stress might be contributing to your pain experience," athletes often hear, "You're weak," or "You're crazy." In other words, they perceive my suggestion as a stereotype threat.

You know what's *really* crazy? The lengths to which some people will go to protect themselves from admitting that they might be vulnerable in this way. I once worked with an athlete named Rachel, whose brother, David, a police officer, suffered from chronic low-back pain. Rachel herself was highly receptive to my biopsychosocial messaging, so she passed some of it along to David in hopes of persuading him to come see me instead of going in for surgery. Alas, David preferred his doctor's diagnosis of a "bad back" to the alternative of a "bad head," which was how he interpreted the suggestion that stress might have a role in his pain experience. So he went ahead and went under the knife, but the doctor operated on the wrong side of his spine, and David was forced to retire from the police force in his 30s.

Lesson learned, right? Nope! David is currently scheduled for a second operation, presumably on the correct side of his back this time.

I don't blame David for the tragedy he willingly walked straight into. The true villain of this story is our culture, which has divorced mind from body so totally that a majority of us either can't comprehend or can't accept the idea that the contents of our head might influence what we feel in our backs or wherever else. Putting blame aside, the whole situation is a damn shame because in rejecting the stress-pain connection, folks like David reject a host of potential pain treatments that are part of stress management.

STRESS MANAGEMENT AS PAIN MANAGEMENT

I don't consider myself an expert on stress management. But I am experienced in considering stress management as a factor in managing pain in athletes, both with the athletes I coach and in my own life. It's pretty simple stuff, really. As jazz great Thelonious Monk said, however, "Simple ain't easy." Effective stress management doesn't happen on its own. It requires consistent, intentional practice of proven measures. In this section, I will discuss the guidance I share most often with athletes with respect to five common stressors: job stress, financial stress, relationship stress, cultural stress, and training stress. Let's tackle the last of these first.

Training Stress

Between 2011 and 2016, the number of reported cases of rhabdomyolysis—a life-threatening condition caused by acute muscle breakdown—increased twentyfold. This sudden explosion in rhabdo-related hospitalizations was a direct result of a meteoric rise in the popularity of CrossFit. Lured by the hardcore ethos of the new exercise craze, thousands of underprepared men and women subjected themselves to workouts far more intense than their bodies were used to—workouts that ravaged their muscles and flooded their blood-streams with biochemical contents that their kidneys had to process.

A small percentage of these victims died of kidney failure. A very large percentage of those who survived their bout with rhabdo—100 percent, in fact—will tell you it hurt like hell. My point in bringing up this unfortunate bit of fitness history is that if you try to train beyond your body's current capacity, you're likely to experience pain. Rhabdo is the most extreme scenario, but even much milder cases of overdoing your training will often generate pain—if not today, then eventually. Avoiding severe pain and injury is not the only reason not to overtrain, of course. Applying more training stress than your body is ready for just isn't a very effective way to get fitter, and getting fitter is, of course, the whole point of training.

The main determinant of how much training is too much is training history. In general, athletes can successfully absorb and adapt to slightly higher levels of training than they've done in the past several weeks. But there are other factors that also influence training capacity, including additional stressors. Remember, you only have one body, and every form of stress affects it. Hence the more stress your body is absorbing outside of your training, the less training you can tolerate. By the same token, the more training you're doing, the less negative stress it takes to push your body beyond its capacity.

The first indicator that your allostatic load has exceeded your body's current adaptive tolerance is fatigue. It's normal to experience fatigue in training, but when it becomes extreme or persistent, something needs to change. Another early sign that your combined training / life stress is excessive is a decline in your motivation to train. As with fatigue, occasional dips in training motivation are normal, but if there's no clear reason for your loss of enthusiasm for working out other than stress, it's very likely that your allostatic load is too great, especially if this emotional symptom is combined with extreme or persistent fatigue.

Experiencing these signs of overload does not necessarily mean pain or injury is just around the corner. The likelihood of these things happening depends on the particulars of your situation and varies among individuals. If you have a history of developing pain in such situations, the chances of a recurrence in similar circumstances are high. The irony is that your awareness of this risk is itself a stressor that could become the proverbial straw that breaks the camel's back. But you can neutralize this factor by reframing it. Instead of thinking of yourself as doomed to get hurt because you're injury-prone, tell yourself that you have a tendency to express high allostatic loads with pain, and to combat this tendency, you need to reduce your stress level and avoid panicking if pain does emerge.

Regardless of your history, if you see signs that your allostatic load is unsustainable, it's important that you take active measures to manage stress. Your first move should be to do anything you can to immediately reduce your life stress. This may spare you from having to reduce your training load. If there's nothing you can do to reduce your life stress right away, then go ahead and back off your training. This is a difficult step to take for many athletes, who associate less training with less fitness. What you need to understand, however, is that in these special circumstances, backing off your training will actually help preserve your fitness. When your allostatic load is high enough that you are persistently fatigued and losing motivation, you're not fully benefiting from your workouts, and you could be on the verge of a pain experience that will *force* you to back off your training or even pause it entirely. A small voluntary training reduction today beats a big involuntary training reduction tomorrow.

Job Stress

Each year, the American Psychological Association conducts a national survey on stress, the results of which are released in a report titled "Stress in America." It probably won't shock you to learn that work is always among the most commonly cited stressors in this survey. Indeed, job stress is so ubiquitous that we tend to assume it's natural and inescapable, but this isn't true. International stress surveys indicate that workers in other countries are not as stressed as American workers, and in some countries, they're significantly less stressed. The American dream is a wonderful thing in many ways, but its pursuit comes at a price.

Does this mean you have no choice but to be frazzled by your efforts to earn a living if you happen to live in the Land of the Rat Race? Of course not. There are plenty of Americans who enjoy manageable levels of work stress. In fact, I'm one of them (most of the time). What's my secret? For starters, I've never cared about money. My ex-father-in-law was a senior vice president at Merrill Lynch, and he just couldn't understand why I wasn't impressed by the original Picasso painting that hung above the toilet in a bathroom in his palatial home. From his perspective, not caring about money was tantamount to not caring about happiness. The funny thing is, for all the money this guy had, I was by far the happier person.

A second reason I experience less work stress than the majority of my fellow Yanks is that I'm not a conformist. I don't aspire to climb the ladder just because others do. When I worked at Coca-Cola, my boss offered me a promotion that I turned down, knowing my path to happiness lay in another direction. When he tried a second time, he got the same answer. Third time too.

The fourth and last time I refused a golden invitation from my boss to scale the corporate ladder, I did so with these words: "Jeff, I've read *Death of a Salesman*, and I'm not interested."

Jeff thought I lacked ambition. He was wrong. I had plenty of ambition for things I was passionate about. Those things just happened to be bouldering and coaching, not job titles and salary increases.

I'm not boasting. Stress gets me too sometimes. My life is not better than yours, and you shouldn't want to be me. But I do have less negative job stress than many people, and having less job stress reduces my risk of experiencing debilitating levels of pain as an athlete. And how I got here is a replicable recipe with three key instructions: (1) Don't let money control your life, (2) Don't make career decisions based on what you think is expected of you, and (3) Do what you love.

As a strength coach—not a life coach—I feel unqualified to tell you what to do with this recipe. The one thing I would insist on is that you do *something* with it. One way or another, use it to claim your power as a working person. Jobs are important, but they're not all that's important. If being an athlete is at all important to you, know that caring a little less about money, doing what feels right instead of always doing what's expected of you, and giving yourself permission to enjoy work will not only help you athletically but also make you happier by reducing the amount of stress in your life. Be conscious of this fact at work tomorrow and the next day. See how it influences your decisions.

Financial Stress

In the most recent "Stress in America" report, financial stress finished in a virtual tie with job stress as the second most commonly experienced stressor. Almost everyone worries about money at one time or another. I know I have. To some extent, candidly, financial stress has been the price I've paid for not prioritizing money in my life. Because I don't care much about money, I've never had a lot of it, and because I've never had a lot of money, I've struggled to make ends meet every now and again.

Interestingly, though, people who place a greater emphasis on money experience just as much financial stress as I do. As the Notorious B.I.G. rapped, "Mo' money, mo' problems." After all, the more you care about something, the more prone you are to stress out about it. If I cared about money just a little bit less than I already do, I would never stress out about it! Also, people (in this country, anyway) tend to adopt a lifestyle that tests the limits of their means regardless of how much money they have. The person who can barely afford to make rent on a crummy studio apartment on skid row is arguably no more stressed out than the person who can barely afford to cover the mortgage on a $50 million estate on Fire Island.

No matter where you stand on the wealth curve, experiencing financial stress will increase your odds of experiencing pain as an athlete. I know this as well as anyone, and you know I know this because I've already told you about how money worries fed into the episode of shoulder pain I experienced when old Butter Bean broke down on Interstate 22 approaching Winfield, Alabama. Other psychological stressors were at play as well, but in hindsight, I do believe that getting past the financial crisis that coincided with the onset of my pain experience helped me get past the pain experience.

I am not a financial adviser, quite obviously, nor do I pretend to be. Heck, I don't even own a suit! In advising you to take measures to reduce the financial stress in your life, my objective is not to set you up for a comfortable retirement and earn a nice commission rate for my trouble. My goal, rather, is to help you experience less training-related pain by keeping your financial stress under control.

There are generally two ways to manage financial stress (or any other stressor, for that matter). One is to change your situation, and the other is to change your attitude toward your situation. Changing your financial situation entails following the advice of experts on personal fiscal responsibility. You've heard this stuff before: Create a realistic household budget, track your spending habits, eliminate wasteful spending, start or continue a saving habit, and so forth. But it's not just your financial situation you can change to reduce stress and pain risk. As an athlete, you can also manipulate your training to work around financial stress. For example, suppose tax season is unavoidably a time of increased financial stress for you each year. In this case, you might choose to plan your training and competition schedule so that you are not pushing your body as hard during tax season and your total allostatic load doesn't become excessive. Save your heaviest training period for the fall, when your financial stress has abated.

When there's not much you can do immediately to improve your financial situation, you can still reduce your financial stress to some extent by changing your attitude toward your situation. Remember that you don't *have to* freak out just because your money is a little tight. When you catch yourself brooding about your financial situation, remind yourself that you've experienced this before and that worrying won't change anything in the meantime. If you have a hard time believing this self-talk, try talking to someone about it.

Relationship Stress

Another common stressor—one that athletes often experience somewhat differently than nonathletes do—is relationship stress. The commitment that athletes make to their sport can be seen by their partners, family members, and close friends as coming at the expense of the relationship. This is especially true when the sport is time-consuming and the athlete is driven to master it. Although I wouldn't say that my passion for climbing was the reason my first marriage didn't work out, it was certainly a source of friction at times, and many of my clients have found themselves in similar positions.

The keys to preventing your athletic pursuits from becoming a source of relationship stress that hinders your athletic pursuits—perhaps by contributing to musculoskeletal pain—are communication and compromise. As the athlete in the relationship, you owe it to your partner, family member, or friend to express that your sport is important to you, and you want to remain committed to it, but your relationship is also important and you are deeply committed to it as well. Ask this person if they can accept your ongoing commitment to athletics and whether they believe it's possible to balance things in a way that makes both of you happy. If the answers to these questions are yes and yes, then all that remains to be done is to negotiate a fair compromise.

I'm aware that the word *negotiate* sounds rather unromantic, but negotiation is a natural part of all close relationships. What happens in too many such relationships is that each party harbors a set of unspoken rules that they want the other to heed, but because the rules are unspoken, they are continually broken. The result is that the same fight keeps repeating over and over again, a Sisyphean pseudonegotiation of hidden agendas. It's much better to make the negotiation explicit, talking through your friction points openly and agreeing to a shared, explicit set of rules.

If the relationship is fundamentally strong, a healthy compromise will be found. Be creative. Many people before you have dealt with the same issue successfully and, in doing so, have come up with all kinds of clever ways to meet in the middle. For example, you might ask your partner to allow you to devote unlimited time to training during a certain part of the year, while you agree to respect a certain time limit the rest of the year. Or you might request permission to build a home-workout room that will allow you to do most of your training within sight of the family. The possibilities are endless, and the potential rewards of identifying the optimal arrangement are great. Healthy, strong relationships are the cornerstone of well-being and hence are ends in themselves, but for athletes, they improve training and potentially lessen pain.

Cultural Stress

And then there's cultural stress—a catchall category that includes everything from social media bullying to politics. This type of stress waxes and wanes over time, but lately, it has been waxing big-time, with all kinds of worrisome stuff happening all at once: pandemics, economic turmoil, climate change and extreme weather events, antidemocratic movements, racial injustice, and the list goes on. In the most recent "Stress in America" survey, the most commonly cited stressor was "the future of America," which to an American sounds perilously close to the end of the world!

One thing I've always noticed is that my stress level goes down when I head to the wilderness for a bouldering project or some other adventure. No doubt the fun I'm having is partly responsible for the drop in blood pressure I experience at these times, but I'm convinced that disconnecting from all the bad stuff that's happening in the world is also a factor. I'm not suggesting that you become disengaged or apathetic for the sake of reducing your allostatic load. You should vote in elections and try to make the world a better place and all that. But what I am suggesting is that you have more power than you might think to buffer yourself from cultural stress.

I know people who have improved their mental health by deleting all their social media accounts. That's a huge step for some, but it's the right step for many. And if it's too big a step for you, there are milder measures you can take, such as filtering out certain content from your feeds and being more selective in what you post, whom you engage with, and how you engage with them.

Turning worry into action is another productive way to deal with cultural stress. Too many of us have passive relationships with the problems of the world, consuming vast amounts of bad news ("doom scrolling") and assuming we're doing our part just by paying attention and caring. In fact, though, this way of engaging with current events neither solves anything nor benefits our mental well-being. If you're concerned about climate change, for example, volunteer for an organization that's committed to combating the problem. Getting involved will release some of the stress surrounding your anxiety about the planet's future and, like the other stress-management measures we've discussed, reduce the impact of pain on your athletic pursuits in the process. The world hasn't ended yet, so you might as well keep looking out for your interests as an athlete!

THE DIAGNOSIS TRAP

Knee pain is common in soccer players. For some, it is a minor nuisance, limiting their play temporarily, and for others, it is highly disruptive, persistently thwarting their ability to enjoy the game they love. A number of factors influence the severity and duration of knee pain in soccer players (or any other type of athlete, for that matter). Among these factors, it may surprise you to learn, is whether a diagnosis is sought. Two former clients of mine, KP and John, both played soccer and both developed knee pain around the same time, but only one of them took the diagnostic route, and that made all the difference—but not in the way most athletes would expect.

KP sought help from a series of clinicians, one of whom, an orthopedic surgeon, diagnosed her with patellofemoral pain syndrome (PFPS), to which she was predisposed on account of her "shitty knees." These were his exact words, as I learned from KP herself, who trained with me for a while between stints under the questionable care of various clinicians. We made a lot of progress in that time—her swelling and pain decreasing markedly and her functional capacity increasing—but not enough to satisfy her, unfortunately. In retrospect, I wish I'd done a better job of communicating to KP that zero pain was not the goal, but this happened several years ago, before my Training as Treatment method had fully matured. As a result, she went further down the therapeutic rabbit hole, trying a litany of modalities, some fringe (postural restoration), others mainstream (dry needling, trigger point therapy), all of them unsupported by science—in search of knees that were less shitty. Alas, KP remains severely limited by knee pain today.

John, meanwhile, took a very different approach to tackling his knee pain. Instead of seeking a medical diagnosis, he started attending group fitness classes at Paragon. His pain level was high enough initially that he walked with a visible hitch in his step, but he did what he could training-wise. A runner as well as a soccer player, he continued to run and play soccer throughout his pain process, reducing his activity level when the knee hurt more and increasing it when it hurt less. I never worked with him one-on-one except to the extent that I give individual attention to all my group-class participants, but John didn't seem to need much guidance. He believed in his ability to feel his way through the process, and he did just that, returning to unlimited practice and play within a few months. When I last checked in with him, John told me his knee was still "grumpy" occasionally, but he's OK with that, as it doesn't stop him from doing what he wants to do.

The point of these two stories should be clear: Getting a concrete diagnosis for a nontraumatic musculoskeletal injury doesn't necessarily accomplish anything, while the effective management of athletic pain does not require a diagnosis. Before I go any further, I should mention that there is a lively debate playing out among physical therapists and others about the value and even the feasibility of nontraumatic musculoskeletal injury diagnosis, and not everyone engaged in it agrees with the statement I just made. That's fine. I'm not trying to win a debate. I'm trying to help athletes minimize the effects of pain on their training and lives, and experience has taught me that in a majority of cases, seeking a diagnosis for athletic pain hinders rather than facilitates successful pain management.

A DIAGNOSIS IS NOT A SOLUTION

Diagnosis is such an integral part of modern medicine that it's easy to forget it didn't always exist. The oldest known reference to the practice appears in an ancient Egyptian medical textbook known as the Edwin Smith Papyrus. Written more than 35 centuries ago, it is believed to be a manual of military surgery, and it stands apart from other medical textbooks of similar vintage in that it attributes wounds, injuries, and other ailments to physical causes and not to spirits or magic.

You wouldn't want to undergo an operation based on the instructions contained in this ancient scroll, naturally. Although ahead of his time, the author was mostly wrong about the physiology of wounds, injuries, and the like. Truly sophisticated medical diagnoses wouldn't become possible until advancements in technology allowed doctors to do more than examine an amputee and say, "Looks like you're missing an arm." Medical historians consider the advent of the stethoscope a watershed moment in this regard. The inventor of this game-changing device was René Laennec, an 18th-century French physician and flutist. Laennec liked to carve his own flutes out of wood, and it was these musical instruments that gave him the inspiration for the medical instrument that has become a symbol of the entire medical profession.

To call the stethoscope revolutionary is no exaggeration, as it enabled doctors, for the first time, to assess the internal health of individuals without reference to how they felt. No longer did patients need to feel something was wrong with them for physicians to know (or believe) something was wrong with them. Many more technologies that did essentially the same thing in different ways followed, so that in historical hindsight, the stethoscope marks the beginning of a modern pivot toward diagnosis-centered medicine, where clinicians place a high priority on identifying health conditions by type, which allows for the best (or most accepted) treatment for each type to be applied.

The stethoscope has saved many lives, as have other diagnostic tools. I have no quarrel with diagnosis as a general practice. What I do have a problem with is the misapplication of this practice. Like any tool, diagnosis is appropriate for some jobs and useless or worse for others. There are certain diseases, rare but treatable, that cannot be properly treated unless they are diagnosed through special tests that represent the 21st-century version of the stethoscope. But sport-related pain is not a rare disease, and the diagnostic impulse to seek the "root cause" of everything does not lead to the best treatment outcomes for athletes experiencing pain that is not associated with acute injury.

Pain Guides the Path to Performance

Pain is inevitable in the life of the athlete. What we all want is to minimize pain's limiting effect on sports participation. Each and every method used to achieve this goal should be judged by a single standard: how effective it really is in minimizing pain's limiting effect on sports participation. Despite what most athletes assume, efforts to diagnose the cause of pain fail miserably by this standard. There are several reasons for this. First and foremost, in a majority of cases, there is nothing to diagnose. It's not that athletes are imagining their pain. Rather, it's that pain does not always signal an injury. More often, pain is just the body's way of letting its limits be known, a kind of organic threat sensor whose sensitivity fluctuates from day to day and situation to situation. Putting the affected body part under the proverbial microscope (or more likely an MRI machine) adds nothing to the message the body communicates internally through pain.

In fact, it's likely to confuse the message. The reason is that when a clinician looks inside the painful part of an athlete's body in search of a cause, there's a good chance they'll find one. And there's an almost equal chance that the cause they find won't be the true or singular cause of the pain. For example, an orthopedist treating a soccer player with persistent knee pain might order an MRI on the knee, and that test might identify a torn meniscus. The orthopedist is then likely to assume the meniscus tear is the cause of the soccer player's pain. But the link between meniscus tears and pain is rather weak. In fact, if you did an MRI on the knees of a young adult with no pain, there's about a 1 in 20 chance you'd find a meniscus tear, and if you did the same thing with an asymptomatic older adult, the odds of finding a tear are 2 in 3.

What Happens When We Get It Wrong?

Misdiagnosis is inherently damaging. An athlete who has been misled about the cause of their pain is less likely to pursue the right solution, which is almost always grounded in strength training and other physical exercise. What's more, misdiagnosis very often leads to other treatments that either don't help or make things worse. Let's go back to our soccer player with knee pain and a torn meniscus. There's a straightforward surgical procedure that is commonly used to fix this injury, and doctors love it because it has a high success rate. But a 2013 study published in the *New England Journal of Medicine* found that patients who underwent a sham meniscus repair surgery were just as likely to get better as those who got the real thing. Musculoskeletal pain has a way of resolving on its own, and it tends to resolve all the more quickly with exercise, but surgeries and other fancy treatments disguise this fact, taking credit they don't deserve for positive outcomes.

As if that wasn't enough, diagnosis has a stigmatizing effect that harms athletes by creating poor expectancies and reducing self-efficacy and also by reinforcing the false notion that pain is caused purely by physical damage. Even when athletes aren't explicitly told they have shitty knees, what they are told has a similar effect. Words often used in diagnosing nontraumatic musculoskeletal injuries—*weak, chronic, imbalance, malalignment, degenerative*—seep into athletes' unconscious, causing them to think of their bodies as abnormal, fragile, unfixable, and ill-suited to the activities they love. As German psychologist Arist von Schlippe summarized, "Descriptions change what is being described."

Reassurance in the Unknown

Defenders of diagnosis like to point out that patients often take comfort in receiving a diagnosis. And they're right. I've lost count of the number of times I've heard an injured athlete say something like "I just wish I knew what it was." But the logic of this justification is circular. The whole reason athletes take comfort in getting a diagnosis is that they've been taught to believe that diagnosis is an essential step toward effective treatment. But as we've just seen, diagnosis is anything but essential to working through athletic pain experiences.

And do you know what's even more comforting than being told the cause of your pain? Knowing you don't *need* to know the cause of your pain! I hear this often as well, specifically from athletes (like John the soccer player) who embrace my Training as Treatment approach and the science it's based on. Believing you can work through your pain experiences on your own or with the help of a coach is reassuring in a way that's superior to believing that receiving a diagnosis takes you one step closer to being fixed by a doctor or physical therapist. That's because the former is a form of belief in yourself, whereas the latter is a form of dependency.

When you truly buy into the idea that you don't need to know what your injury is called and that it's probably not even an injury, you experience far less worry and uncertainty the next time pain comes calling. And unlike having confidence in medical diagnoses, this inner confidence won't let you down. If you act on the belief that you can work through your pain independently, the outcome will validate this belief, as happened for John. But when you put your faith in diagnosis and in diagnosis-based treatments, you're more likely to end up like KP, with nothing to show for all the time spent in clinicians' offices except a bunch of labels attached to your pain.

A NEW APPROACH TO INJURY

What is an injury, anyway? It's quite easy to give examples of injuries yet surprisingly difficult to come up with a definition of *injury* that's capable of withstanding scrutiny. The boundaries are always smudgy, blurred by examples that don't quite fit. Is a bruise an injury if it was caused by sepsis or a bleeding disorder rather than by impact with a foreign object? Is a cut an injury if it was caused by a surgeon's scalpel? Is a muscle tear an injury if the torn muscle still functions normally? Is a pinched nerve an injury?

I have no interest in coming up with my own definition of *injury*. Instead, I prefer simply to use the word as sparingly as possible. If I were a paramedic whose job was to pull accident victims out of wrecked cars, I wouldn't be so reticent. But as a strength coach, I don't think the word *injury* applies to most of the conditions it is commonly applied to in athletes. Tissue damage is considered a defining feature of injury, but how much damage must exist in a muscle, bone, or connective tissue before it qualifies as injured? Enough to cause dysfunction, certainly. But then how much dysfunction must exist in a damaged tissue before we slap the injury label on it? The day after you complete a marathon, there's muscle damage in your legs, and you have trouble descending stairs. Are you injured?

Heck, even after a single bout of strength training, your muscles are damaged, and it's likely you'll also be sore and have reduced functional capacity. But fast-forward a day or two, and your muscles are actually stronger than they were before the workout because they've adapted to the stress it imposed. Our bodies aren't just resilient; they're antifragile—in other words, they can not only withstand stress and the damage and pain that are often associated with it but *depend* on these things to adapt and improve. All of which makes it really hard to know what is and isn't an injury.

None of this would matter if words didn't have power, but words do have power, and overusing the word *injury* does a lot of harm that can be avoided by limiting its application to cases where it's strictly necessary. An athlete who says, "My knee hurts," is not merely speaking differently than an athlete who says, "My knee is injured." That athlete is also *thinking* differently, and because they're thinking differently, they're likely to act differently as well. While the athlete who speaks of injury stops training for fear of causing more damage and seeks outside help, the athlete who speaks only of pain keeps training, albeit with sensible modifications, and avoids depending on others for a successful outcome.

The word *injury* isn't exactly verboten at Paragon Athletics, but you won't hear it very often, especially from athletes who've been working with me for a while. It's amazing to see how their whole mindset toward pain shifts as their use of the word dwindles. Try banishing the word *injury* from your vocabulary for a while, and see if it doesn't lead to a deeper change—one you won't regret.

INJURIES THAT AREN'T INJURIES

At Paragon, I practice an informal version of what is known as *dediagnosing*, which has been defined by Marianne Lea and Bjorn Morten Hofmann of the University of Oslo as "*the removal of diagnoses that do not contribute to reducing the person's suffering,* i.e., when the person is better off without it." It works like this: Athletes come to me having been diagnosed with an injury that has no value in being diagnosed, and I reverse that diagnosis—not by telling them they're not really injured but by *showing* them. What follows are three examples of common injury diagnoses that are particularly problematic. I present them with the intent of driving home the point that true injury of the nonacute type is relatively rare in sports and of encouraging you to stop saying you're injured, thinking you're injured, and acting like you're injured unless you truly are injured by *anyone's* definition.

Rotator Cuff Tear

When I think about rotator cuff tears, the first person who comes to mind is Roxanna Brock McDade, a world-class climber based here in Flagstaff. Some time ago, Roxanna was diagnosed with a full-thickness tear of her supraspinatus, one of four muscles that make up the rotator cuff. Certain functional tests, including the "painful arc test" (what a name!), which entails lifting the arm out to the side and up overhead, are commonly used in making this diagnosis, but they are pitifully unreliable—and that's not just my opinion. In 2020, the *Journal of Orthopaedic & Sports Physical Therapy* published a viewpoint that posed the question, "Is It Time to Put Special Tests for Rotator Cuff-Related Pain Out to Pasture?" The four-page article can be summarized in a single word: "yes."

There are both conservative treatments (physical therapy) and aggressive treatments (surgery) for full-thickness rotator cuff tears. Roxanna's doctor started her off with the former, but despite being a model physical therapy patient, she made little progress. I see this all too often. Even elite-level athletes like Roxanna are set up to fail when they are given a devastating diagnosis, labeled a patient, and placed in therapy. The whole process sets low expectations that, in Roxanna's case and in so many others, are largely self-fulfilling. A 2016 study appearing in the *Journal of Shoulder and Elbow Surgery* reported that within a group of 433 individuals diagnosed with full-thickness rotator cuff tears, a low outcome expectation for physical therapy was the strongest predictor of who ended up having surgery.

After physical therapy failed, Roxanna was brought back in for medical imaging—specifically an MRI—which confirmed the existence of tissue disruption extending straight through the supraspinatus muscle. Roxanna now had one last chance to avoid surgery, and that chance was me. We worked together for several weeks, during which period her pain level decreased significantly while her ability to use the shoulder increased commensurately. She moved up the ladder from phase 1 exercises to phase 2 exercises to phase 3 exercises, and then she graduated to self-directed training.

Later, Roxanna sent me an email message with a large file attached. "Check this out," she wrote. The attachment was an image from a follow-up MRI, which showed no tear. To be clear, rotator cuff tears do heal, but not that quickly. Roxanna's supraspinatus hadn't been torn in the first place, or at least not as badly as she'd been told.

The risk of misdiagnosis and the psychological trauma that it can cause are not the only reasons athletes should avoid seeking a diagnosis for shoulder pain not associated with an acute incident. Another reason is that the existence of tissue damage in the rotator cuff doesn't really tell us anything useful. A 2019 study by Brazilian researchers makes this point quite clearly. A group of 123 individuals experiencing pain in one shoulder had MRIs done on both of their shoulders—the one that hurt and the one that didn't. The results? Structural damage was nearly as common on the pain-free side as on the painful side.

This doesn't mean tissue damage has nothing to do with shoulder pain. But it's never more than a piece of the story, and in the vast majority of cases, finding damage in the rotator cuff of a person with shoulder pain has no practical relevance to their getting better. Whether a person with shoulder pain has damage or no damage in the rotator cuff or somewhere else, the way to get better is to use the shoulder within acceptable pain limits, challenging it more and more as those limits are pushed back, while also addressing possible psychological or social contributors to the pain experience, such as allostatic load and lack of pain self-efficacy.

By the way, everything I've just said about rotator cuff tears applies to other nontraumatic shoulder injuries. Indeed, when you give up on trying to identify a singular physical cause of shoulder pain, all the different labels used to distinguish one injury from another disappear. As far back as 2008, Dutch researchers argued for doing precisely this, writing, "We strongly suggest [that we] abolish the use of these labels and direct future research towards undivided populations with 'general' shoulder pain."

Where is your pain located? How much does it hurt? What can you do with it, and what can't you do? Your answers to these questions are the only diagnosis you need.

Nonspecific Low-Back Pain

Shoulder pain and low-back pain have a lot in common. But one of the ways they're different is that doctors have a somewhat easier time finding a specific damaged muscle, tendon, or other tissue to blame for pain in the shoulder than they do for pain in the low back. In fact, it is estimated that in only 8 to 15 percent of cases are efforts to identify a specific anatomical "cause" of low-back pain successful. Hence the term *nonspecific low-back pain*, which is a kind of catchall nondiagnosis used to label the vast majority of low-back pain sufferers who don't appear to have anything particularly wrong in their spine.

Because pathoanatomy is seldom the primary cause of low-back pain (and never the singular cause), the very attempt to find a damaged structure to blame for low-back pain violates the first principle of the Hippocratic oath ("First, do no harm"), as science writer Paul Ingraham argues in an article for *Pain Science*, writing, "You simply cannot reliably diagnose low back pain with MRI or with X-ray in isolation—and trying to do so reliably raises false alarms that actually *do harm*. Premature MRI is actually often *worse* than useless, scaring patients badly."

What's more, the results of imaging done on people with low-back pain often have a negative biasing effect on both patient and physician. Proof of this comes from a study conducted by Indian scientists and published in the *European Spine Journal* in 2021. A group of 44 individuals with low-back pain underwent an MRI scan, after which half of them were given a factual description of the findings and half were told that the findings were normal regardless of the results. Six weeks later, according to the study's authors, members of the first group had a "more negative perception of their spinal condition, increased catastrophization, decreased pain improvement, and poorer functional status." What's more, in a separate part of the same study, two different sets of terminology were used to present MRI results to clinicians who were given no other information about the patients. One set included commonly used catastrophizing language, such as "degeneration," while the other was scrubbed of such language. Clinicians rated the same individual cases as less severe and recommended less extreme treatment measures when the results were presented without the usual negative bias.

As with shoulder pain, I'm not suggesting that tissue disruption is a nonfactor in low-back pain. But research has clearly demonstrated that structural damage is just one of many factors, as Peter O'Sullivan of Curtin University pointed out in a paper titled "It's Time for Change with the Management of Non-specific Chronic Low Back Pain," stating, "There is strong evidence that NSCLBP disorders are associated with a complex combination of physical, behavioral, lifestyle, neuro-physiological (peripheral and central nervous system changes), psychological/cognitive and social factors. These factors together have the potential to promote maladaptive cognitive behaviors (negative beliefs, fear, avoidance, catastrophizing, hypervigilance), pain behaviors (pain communicative and avoidant behaviors) and movement behaviors, setting up a vicious cycle of pain sensitization and reinforcing disability."

Despite overwhelming evidence that pathoanatomy is seldom the main cause of low-back pain and that magic-bullet treatments such as spinal injections and disc replacements are ineffective, doctors continue to diagnose single causes of low-back pain and treat its physical dimension in isolation from its other dimensions. As a strength coach, I couldn't treat low-back pain in these ways if I wanted to, but even if I could, I wouldn't because I believe what the science plainly tells us.

Recently, I worked with an athlete who, without intending to, forced me to put up or shut up concerning my belief in the biopsychosocial nature of low-back pain. A renowned orthopedic surgeon, Peter referred himself to me for help with persistent low-back pain despite being a confirmed believer in the structuralist model of athletic injury that I abandoned years ago. He had already undergone one back surgery and was scheduled for a second procedure to relieve a compressed sciatic nerve when he came to me. I suppose Peter was just desperate enough to give my way a try before he went back under the knife.

Sciatic nerve compression is a real phenomenon, though it is far more rare than people think, existing only in low-back pain sufferers who also exhibit severe neurological signs, including weakness and atrophy in the legs. Peter had none of these signs, and while he believed that nerve compression told the whole story of his low-back pain, I felt equally certain that such structural issues are never more than part of the story. And here again, I have science on my side, as research has consistently shown that psychosocial factors play an especially big role in low-back pain. To give just one example, around the time I started helping Peter, the journal *Nature* published a study on the association between low-back pain and general life stress. The study's authors compared stress levels in a group of individuals with chronic low-back pain and a group without it. Here's what they found:

Study on Association Between Chronic Low-Back Pain and Life Stress

	LOW-BACK PAIN GROUP	NO LOW-BACK PAIN GROUP
Percent reporting severe stress	6.66	3.55
Percent reporting moderate stress	23.40	13.73
Percent reporting mild stress	50.60	57.11
Percent reporting no stress	19.34	25.61

As you can see, individuals reporting moderate to high levels of general life stress were far more likely to experience chronic low-back pain in this large sample. Granted, there is no proof of causality here, but we know from other research that the causal link between stress and pain goes in both directions, so even if some of the general life stress reported by low-back pain sufferers was caused by their discomfort, we can be confident that stress was also a contributing factor in their pain experience.

Peter had more than his share of general life stress at the time he developed low-back pain. In addition to holding an extremely demanding job with tremendous responsibility, he was the husband of a woman with stage 4 cancer and the father of a son with a substance-abuse problem. Knowing this, I decided early on to focus on Peter himself rather than on his low back. None of the exercises we did together targeted the low back specifically, and we did a lot more talking than exercising during his visits to the gym. After all, this was a man who spent all day every day taking care of others, and I felt that more than anything else, he just needed someone to take care of him for a change. I believe my work with Peter did help in the sense that it gave him a healthy opportunity to put his well-being first and it kept him active. It did not help his pain symptoms, however, and Peter went ahead with the second procedure, which also didn't help.

It's unfortunate that neither my gym work with Peter nor surgery ameliorated his low-back pain. But it also validated my hunch that life stress was a major contributor to it, as that's the one thing that didn't change in all of this. He still comes to Paragon regularly for group fitness classes, though, and I'm happy about that.

Achilles Tendinopathy

Among the athletes who come to my gym having already been diagnosed with an injury, a plurality have been told they have tendonitis. This is not surprising. There are tendons all over the body, and it's hard to find a sport that doesn't subject one or more tendons to high levels of repetitive stress. In climbers, the elbow is the most common site of tendon-centered pain, and in runners, it's the Achilles.

Tendonitis is by no means the only tendon injury. Researchers are working hard to perfect the system by which tendon injuries are classified and diagnosed. Among the factors considered in classifying tendon injuries are the location of tissue disruption (insertional vs. midportion) and whether it is reactive (i.e., leading to repair) or degenerative. It is assumed by many of the experts who are involved in this classification effort that once they've got all the terminology nailed down, patients will be more precisely diagnosed and more effectively treated, but I have my doubts. As with other injuries and so-called injuries, the link between symptoms and tissue disruption is rather loose in tendonitis and other tendon injuries. This was shown in a study led by Kevin Lieberthal of Australian Catholic University and published in *Physical Therapy in Sport* in 2019. A group of 37 distance runners who had never experienced Achilles tendon pain underwent ultrasound imaging. Nearly half of these individuals had "abnormalities" in at least one tendon that were significant enough to have been blamed for any pain the runners felt in that area. Findings like these suggest that learning more about the various tissue changes that occur in tendons is unlikely to help athletes better manage tendon pain.

In the meantime, we know that strength training works quite well to manage tendon pain by changing the tissues involved through multiple pathways, reducing inhibition through exposure, provoking an immune response, and increasing self-efficacy. Athletes who use the Training as Treatment approach to address tendon pain often improve a lot faster than the affected tissue itself could possibly respond. I encourage my athletes not to worry about what's going on underneath their skin, explaining that the process isn't about reducing inflammation or promoting healing or anything of that nature. We're just tinkering around with different ways of using the tendon and leaning into their pain at a level that's acceptable to them, taking what we can get until pain no longer prevents them from doing everything they want to do.

All too commonly, athletes who seek a diagnosis for tendon pain are either told to rest or sent to a physical therapist who, instead of training them, places them in therapy, which is only slightly better than rest. I once worked with a motocross racer who was told by a doctor to rest his injured elbow until the pain went away completely, which could take up to two years. During this period of doctor-prescribed sedentariness, he gained 20 pounds, became depressed, and saw no improvement in symptoms. Then he came to Paragon. Together, we were able to reverse these consequences of inactivity, though not right away. To avoid a similar experience, don't seek a diagnosis the next time you experience tendon-centered pain associated with exercise.

WHEN DIAGNOSIS IS APPROPRIATE

One fine winter's day, my friend Tim slipped and fell on a patch of black ice while running, landing on his right side. Not surprisingly, his ribs hurt the next morning. But when his ribs still hurt several weeks later, Tim was more than just surprised—he was concerned. That's when he called me to ask for my advice. I assured Tim that it's quite normal for pain associated with even minor rib injuries to take its sweet time in going away and that he should brace for a lengthy process. Even I was surprised, though, when instead of slowly improving over the next couple of months, Tim's rib pain got even worse. Long story short, Tim finally went in for imaging and discovered that a benign tumor was growing in his rib cage, right where he'd landed. It was a coincidence, of course—the tumor had nothing whatsoever to do with whatever damage he'd sustained, but it had everything to do with his pain experience.

The lesson here is that sometimes, it is wise to seek a diagnosis for a pain experience. While Tim's rib pain was a one-in-a-million fluke, and my intent in sharing his story is not to cause you to worry that your next sore spot might be tumorous, there are a few more common pain scenarios that signal something other than everyday pain and warrant medical attention.

As I've mentioned previously, acute injuries are categorically different from pain experiences not associated with a single event. If you're out training and you suffer a fall, hear a snap, or feel something suddenly give way and intense pain ensues, you should consult a physician. Also, remember the red-flag scenarios that were enumerated in Chapter 8. If, in addition to pain, you experience numbness or weakness, incontinence, or significant bruising or swelling, deformation, seizure, loss of consciousness, confusion, or a "gut feeling" that something's not right, call a doctor. Additionally, whenever pain is severe enough to interfere not only with your normal training but also with activities of daily living such as carrying groceries and getting into and out of your car, it's worth getting checked out.

Outside of these scenarios, there are only a handful of injuries and conditions that you can't train through without a diagnosis or medical intervention. Stress fractures are one. If your pain seems to be centered in a bone and you've had a recent spike in your training load or adopted a restrictive diet, I recommend having it looked at. I'm keenly conscious of the fact that I've listed enough exceptions to my general caution against seeking diagnosis to give the worriers license to see a doctor for every pain experience "just to be safe." But keep in mind, seeking a diagnosis is not harmless, and the vast majority of pain experiences not associated with acute trauma do not require it.

11

LEAVING THE NEST

Congratulations! You've made it to the final chapter. I'm not being glib; you now have a solid understanding of the core principles of the biopsychosocial model of pain as the basis for my belief that athletes generally can and should manage their sports-related pain experiences (the vast majority of which do not qualify as injuries) without the help of medical professionals. If you still have some doubt, that's understandable too. Although I've since gotten used to it, I was initially shocked by how difficult it is to get these ideas to penetrate the thinking of doctors, physical therapists, and other clinicians who treat (but don't train) athletes with pain. That these same ideas appear to have penetrated your own thinking is a good thing, but it is not without consequences. What's good is that you will no longer be as dependent on medical professionals as you were before. The consequence of this is that, being a step ahead of the medical professionals, you may no longer feel you can depend on them (or anyone else, for that matter) to help you navigate your way through pain experiences. And unless you are already confident that you can navigate these situations on your own, this new state of independence might seem a bit scary, like being pushed out of the nest before you're ready (or at least before you feel you're ready), forced to fly on untested wings.

The purpose of this concluding chapter is to equip you for your first solo flight in the atmosphere of Training as Treatment. Learning to manage your pain doesn't mean that you will be completely on your own. There are people who can help guide you through a version of Training as Treatment whenever pain intrudes on your training. I am one of them—you can always find me at paragonathletics.com—and I will show you how to find other like-minded coaches. But first, I must do like Momma Bird and give you a final push out of the nest so you can more effectively minimize the impact of pain on your athletic performance.

A BATTLE OF BELIEF

Greg Lehman's visit to Paragon Athletics in 2017, which I first mentioned in Chapter 5, was an eye-opening experience for me. But it wasn't his message itself that opened my eyes. Rather, it was the failure of his message to connect with the 50 or so physical therapists and other clinicians who attended the two-day course on Reconciling Biomechanics with Pain Science.

During the breakout sessions on day two, Greg presented to the group a series of hypothetical cases and asked us how we would handle them. Each of these scenarios involved a pain presentation that, as Greg well knew, lacked a standard treatment protocol. The one that stands out in my memory was an athlete with anterior hip pain. Greg invited the members of the group to share ideas about how to work with this individual, and because all of them used standard treatment protocols exclusively when treating pain, they were at a complete loss as to what to suggest.

"Uh, squats?" someone ventured.

As luck would have it, I was at that time working with an athlete who was scheduled for surgery to fix a femoroacetabular impingement (FAI), which is a fancy term for anterior hip pain, so I explained the approach I was taking with this athlete. Even if I'd lacked this concrete example, however, I could have described the approach I would have taken with such a person, because I don't use standard treatment protocols with anyone. The real advantage I had over my fellow breakout group members was that I understood pain does not equal injury, and I knew how to use exercise to manage pain, whereas clinicians are taught that they need to identify the specific injury underlying a pain presentation to treat it properly. Because most clinicians are not schooled in the basics of strength and conditioning, they are ill-equipped to use exercise effectively to manage pain.

When Greg's course wrapped up that same afternoon, I went around the room asking each attendee what they'd thought of it. To my dismay, nearly all of them gave no indication of being open to the message of pain science. These were highly educated medical professionals, after all, and as such they all believed they had indeed understood the course. But insofar as they had understood it, they'd done so through misinterpretation, assimilating Greg's antistructuralist message into their existing structuralist understanding of pain and injury. Whereas Greg had taught them that treatment protocols don't work because they're based on a false premise, they had learned that they might need to tweak their protocols a bit—but then again, maybe not, because who does this Greg Lehman guy think he is, anyway?

People tend to believe what they want to believe, and what they want to believe is what they perceive to be in their interest to believe. To draw an analogy, you'd be hard-pressed to find a wealthy economist who doesn't believe in supply-side economic theory, which proposes that everyone in society, from the richest to the poorest, benefits most when policy is tailored to serve the short-term profit interests of the richest. Now, supply-side theory might be true, but if it is (and it isn't), that's not why wealthy economists believe it's true. Similarly, medical professionals who treat athletes benefit from believing that pain equals injury and that only trained medical professionals are qualified to treat injuries. In my mind, Greg's performance at Paragon Athletics nullified this doctrine as overwhelmingly as Nobel Prize–winning economist Paul Krugman's work nullified supply-side economics, but what matters on a practical level, unfortunately, is not what's true but who has the power.

CAUSE FOR HOPE

I'm aware of how cynical this sounds, but I promise you, I'm no cynic. More often than not, I believe, truth prevails in the end, despite the impediments. This is especially likely in practical domains such as sports and exercise, where truth and results are closely linked and results carry the day. When I first got into bouldering, for example, many top climbers believed the only training they needed was climbing itself. But I happened to believe that supplemental strength training could improve performance and reduce pain and injury, and because my belief happened to be true, it yielded better results, and today (not entirely due to my influence, of course) most top climbers strength train regularly.

I'm confident that Training as Treatment will prove to be the best path to performance for athletes. I can't predict how it will happen or how long it will take, but I've seen some promising signs, one of which came on the very same day I realized what Training as Treatment was up against. There was, in fact, one person who attended Greg's course on Reconciling Biomechanics with Pain Science and emerged with a new perspective: my friend Jenny, herself a physical therapist. She explained to me that embracing Greg's message would require most professionals to largely give up on diagnosing and treating injuries and focus instead on training their clients (whom they should no longer regard as patients), reducing them to glorified personal trainers—a demotion, from their perspective. But Jenny herself didn't feel this way, and if one physical therapist could embrace Training as Treatment, I figured others could too.

It was also Jenny who steered me toward Eric Malzone, a fitness industry entrepreneur who advises other entrepreneurs in the industry, which I suppose I am. One thing led to another, and I soon found myself delivering my own version of Greg's message, grounded in the work we were doing at Paragon, on Eric's podcast. "We've earned a reputation for helping people through musculoskeletal issues," I told him during that interview. "Very often those folks have been passed through the medical system. Thankfully, we've had a lot of success stories, and like I say, it's earned us a reputation for being able to help folks get over the hump. Probably 50 percent of my day is devoted to helping those athletes, and the other 50 percent is just training folks. But we don't see a difference between the two, and we don't think they should be seen as different." In the moment, I couldn't tell whether, like Jenny, Eric got it. But it turned out he did—so much so that Eric subsequently invited me to create an online course that would teach Training as Treatment to other professionals. I jumped at the opportunity, seeing it as a way to hasten the revolution that I believe needs to happen.

The purpose of the course is to equip strength coaches, personal trainers, and yes, physical therapists, with the knowledge and skills they need to do what I do at Paragon Athletics. My hope is that, eventually, the program trains enough practitioners to serve the needs of every athlete who wants professional help in training through pain. Notice I said "wants," not "needs." I stand by my claim that athletes are capable of self-managing pain related to their sport. But that doesn't mean athletes can't benefit from working with a coach, trainer, or physical therapist. At a minimum, these professionals can help athletes who are new to Training as Treatment build confidence as they begin proactively managing their pain. Beyond that, though, I don't deny that a true specialist—who knows their science, pays their dues in education and training, and gains broad experience in helping athletes with pain—can make the process of training through pain more efficient than it might otherwise be, particularly for an athlete who is also new to strength training.

In this respect, Training as Treatment is no different from training as most athletes know it. The world's simplest sport, arguably, is long-distance running, whose repetitive nature brings me a lot of clients. And history's greatest long-distance runner, arguably, is Eliud Kipchoge, the Kenyan legend who twice won the Olympic marathon and twice broke the marathon world record. Yet despite the simplicity of long-distance running, and despite his greatness, Kipchoge chose throughout his unparalleled career to work with a coach, Patrick Sang. Kipchoge said in one interview that Sang "knows how to make an athlete a normal human being and a star at the same time."

My point is that good coaches are valuable, even when they are not strictly needed. That is why I'm trying to do my part to make good coaching available to every athlete who wants help training through pain. Even in the best-case scenario, however, it's going to take time to educate and train an adequate supply of such professionals. The good news is that I'm not the only qualified person working to change how professionals handle pain and performance.

HOW TO FIND PROFESSIONAL SUPPORT

Even now, there are lots of coaches, trainers, and even some physical therapists who practice something approximating Training as Treatment. In fact, these professionals have always existed. They regard pain as normal, distinguish pain from injury, take a collaborative approach to working with athletes who have pain, are careful to avoid making clients feel fragile or stuck, believe that athletes can train through most pain experiences, and have a record of success in doing so. But how do you identify these folks?

Start by asking your fellow athletes if they work with, have worked with, or know of a coach or trainer who's good at helping athletes avoid and overcome injuries. (Admittedly, it's really pain and not "injuries" you are inquiring about.) If your training buddies aren't able to point you in the right direction, try posing the same question on online athlete forums or posting an open social media callout.

The next step is to do your due diligence on the coaches, trainers, or therapists you're led to through your search. You might ask if they are familiar with *Pain and Performance* and whether they agree with its message. You can also grill your prospective coach or trainer about their experience with "injured" athletes, what their approach is to training such athletes, and what their beliefs are about how to prevent and manage injuries. You might even ask for a reference or two—ideally, a current or past client they've helped through injury.

Remember, while some of the science that informs Training as Treatment is new, most of its core principles and methods are not. Indeed, to a great extent, my approach is a return to old ways. In practical terms, what this means for you as an athlete who's looking for good coaching is that you'll have a better chance of getting it from old-school types. Prior to the medicalization of athletic pain, coaches and trainers didn't send athletes to the sports medicine clinic every time they felt a niggle somewhere. Instead, they helped athletes manage pain experiences (not resulting from acute injury) by making sensible modifications to their training. Such coaches and trainers still exist. They tend to be the ones who work out of nondescript facilities that lack mirrors on the walls and machines of any kind. They are also the ones who give you the same advice on nutrition, sleep, and fresh air that your grandmother gave you when you were a kid. They spend a lot more time asking athletes how their workout felt than they do analyzing data captured by some fancy wearable device. Their knowledge of exercise science is current, but they don't go chasing after every new trend that comes along.

The better coaches and trainers out there also respect and address the psychological and social dimensions of pain. They may never refer to the biopsychosocial model, but experience has taught them that being an athlete is not just an activity a person engages in but a part of their identity. As a result, they take measures to preserve this sense of identity when working with athletes experiencing pain, for example, by keeping them active and around other athletes. They also understand the relevance of stress and emotion to training and performance and will do what they can within their role to keep an athlete's enjoyment level high and stress in check as they work through a pain experience, through measures such as involving them in decision-making and being a listening ear when they just need to talk.

In saying all this, I don't mean to give you the impression that you need a coach. Most of the success stories I've shared with you involve athletes who no longer work with me, yet they are able to manage pain effectively on their own based on what they learned. I simply help athletes get past their immediate problem *and* instill in them the knowledge and skills they need to manage future pain experiences on their own. You now possess this same foundation, and you are now as ready to leave the nest as any of my in-person clients.

NAVIGATING YOUR OWN PAIN AND PERFORMANCE

In September 2021, I suffered a freak mishap while playing around on the climbing wall at Paragon. I had reached a stopping point and let go of the wall, intending to drop down to the crash mat below as I'd done a million times before. But just then, a fleck of chalk found its way into my left eye, distracting me for a critical split second and causing my right foot to land on the edge of the mat and roll outward in a way that no foot ever should. The pain was intense, but being who I am, I rested for only one day before starting the process of training my way back to symptom resolution and full function. Within two months, I was doing single-leg box jumps and wind sprints—mission accomplished. Or so I thought.

My next big climbing trip took me to Joshua Tree. On the morning we left, I spent two hours sitting cross-legged on a sofa, reading Dan Cleather's *Force: The Biomechanics of Training*. When I tried to stand up, I couldn't put weight on my right foot. The pain was back, as intense as ever. Canceling the trip was unthinkable, yet climbing was unimaginable, so I spent the first day in Joshua Tree gimping around as though I was walking on broken glass with one shoe off. Observing my hobbled state, my friend Jason, who was belaying his wife, Susan, at the time, asked me what had happened, and I told him. He seemed unsurprised.

"I've been there," he said, dividing his attention between Susan, who was cleaving to a rock face twenty feet above us, and me. "It's been my experience that aggravated joint tissues don't like stretching. They like loading. If I were you, I'd start putting that ankle under load as soon as you can. It'll get better faster that way."

Mind you, Jason is not an orthopedist or a physical therapist or even a trainer, but he has spent much of his life participating in two sports—ultrarunning and climbing—that are pretty darn tough on the body. He's self-reliant by nature and has figured out how to competently manage athletic pain on his own, just as I did as a young boulderer before I went down the rabbit hole of sports medicine and physical therapy.

Athletes like Jason are living proof that it's possible to manage athletic pain on your own. Sure, Jason happens to know me personally, but there are also many athletes who intuit the core principles and methods of Training as Treatment without so much as knowing that I exist. Remember my father-in-law, Jim? He hurt his shoulder falling off a horse and recovered fully without anyone's help. And don't forget about Matt, my writing partner, who discovered a number of the truths expressed in this book through his own trial and error. It's my hope that *Pain and Performance* empowers athletes to work through pain experiences more efficiently and assuredly. When Jim hurt his shoulder a second time, he recovered a lot quicker by employing the Training as Treatment method, and as Matt reported in his introduction, the knowledge he took away from my "Pain and Performance" presentation helped him manage his future pain experiences even more effectively. You can do the same.

When I came home from my trip to Joshua Tree, I contacted my friend Steve, an orthopedist who lives and practices in Mammoth Lakes, California. The setback I'd experienced with my ankle two months after I twisted it was surprising enough that I felt the need to get a trusted outsider's perspective on it. Steve and I go back a ways; I've trained him and his wife, who is an elite athlete herself, for years, and he often refers patients to me. I use Steve as a sounding board whenever I find myself a bit out of my depth with an athlete, and this time that athlete was me.

I told Steve about the climbing wall incident and the setback precipitated by sitting quietly at home with a book. As always, Steve listened patiently, asked thoughtful questions, showed genuine empathy, and wasn't too quick to draw conclusions or tell me what to do. He did, however, put forward the possibility that instead of rupturing a ligament in my ankle, as I suspected, I had chipped a bone, loosening a fragment that had slid into a gap in the joint that opened while I was sitting cross-legged, angering the surrounding tissues when I put weight on the foot. In the end, we agreed to give the situation more time to resolve itself. If after six weeks I was still dealing with a lot of pain, we'd look at other options, including exploratory surgery.

I know what you're thinking: "You've convinced me not to call the doctor when I experience pain related to my sport. And now here you are calling the doctor after experiencing pain related to your sport! What gives?" That's a fair question. But here's the thing: My goal is to put you in control of your athletic pain experiences. That's it. And it so happens that taking control of their pain experiences requires most athletes to become less reliant on doctors than they currently are. But when you are in control of your pain experiences, you can use doctors as an additional pain-management tool when necessary without ceding control to them, and there are some doctors out there who genuinely want you to remain in control—and Steve is one of them.

And while we're at it, let's not forget that Greg Lehman, who works as a physiotherapist, is the professional that is perhaps more responsible than any other for restoring the control of pain management to athletes. If you were to seek Greg's help in dealing with a particular pain experience, you can be sure he wouldn't subject you to unreliable diagnostic tests or use language that caused you to feel fragile and to fear movement. In short, just as Steve is living proof that there are doctors capable of working with, rather than against, your efforts to practice Training as Treatment, Greg Lehman is living proof that there are also some physical therapists who are capable of doing the same. But how do you identify them?

CONSULTING CLINICIANS

The main thing to look for in a sports medicine doctor or physical therapist is a so-called patient-centered (I prefer "person-centered") approach to care. This means that in each interaction you have with him or her, the clinician shows empathy and humility, is patient with you, listens attentively, takes you seriously, seems to genuinely care about your well-being, is open-minded and willing to experiment, and takes a collaborative approach to helping you achieve your desired outcomes. The initial intake process should feel natural rather than formal, and the clinician should ask questions that go beyond your symptoms and history, creating a human context around the problem that brought you to the clinician's office.

If you can find a clinician who has these qualities and a background in strength and conditioning, so much the better. Among physical therapists, this is reasonably common, but among doctors, not so much. The best alternative to a clinician with comprehensive training and deep experience in strength and conditioning is one whose practice is focused on athletes or who has a strong relationship with one or more local coaches and trainers to whom they refer athletes, as Steve does with me. It doesn't hurt if the clinician is also an athlete.

I will say one last time for the record that you should consult medical professionals only in red-flag scenarios or when your efforts to manage a pain experience alone or with a coach or trainer aren't succeeding. And when you do reach out to a doctor or physical therapist, be selective, using the criteria I've just given you to separate the few clinicians who "get it" from the many who don't. The research required to do this might seem onerous, but it's worthwhile.

There's no shame, by the way, in wanting to put yourself in the hands of an expert when you're experiencing pain. It's human nature to seek help when facing challenges. You probably could fix a leaky faucet in your home without help if you put your mind to it, but you might prefer to pay a professional plumber to take care of it for you. Pain experiences are no different. Why face them alone when someone else can help you negotiate them? As you've learned, however, no expert—regardless of how knowledgeable and experienced they are—can truly handle your pain experiences for you. Yet the better coaches and trainers know this, so you can really have it both ways. If a part of you still wishes some expert *could* handle your pain for you, go ahead and find a coach or trainer (or therapist) who meets the requirements I've articulated. That person will then promptly set about the business of guiding you through your present pain experience in a way that prepares you to be more independent—and confident—the next time around. You can do this! You'll see.

Oh, by the way, my ankle injury turned out to be one of the most mysterious injuries I've ever had. Also keep in mind it was an acute injury, involving significant trauma to all ligaments, tendons, and soft tissues surrounding my ankle. However, I am happy to say that after many confusing months and a lot of consistent training, I am back to being able to focus on climbing and not the potential for pain. Stay the course.

Appendix

The end of this book is the beginning of your personal practice of the Training as Treatment method. Use the link that follows to access video demonstrations of exercises we often use with clients at Paragon Athletics. They are grouped according to the area of the body they target (feet and ankles, knees, hips, shoulders, and low back) and the phase of the process (1–3) where they best fit.

Being in pain is not a requirement for incorporating these exercises into your training and benefiting from them. Remember that there is no need to differentiate between training and treatment—treatment is just training in the presence of pain. As you get stronger and/or your pain diminishes, follow the progression guidelines offered in Chapter 7 to keep moving forward. You can request a consultation with one of the trainers at Paragon if you have questions.

References

Introduction

Babatunde OO, Jordan JL, Van der Windt DA, Hill JC, Foster NE, Protheroe J. Effective treatment options for musculoskeletal pain in primary care: A systematic overview of current evidence. *PLOS One.* 2017 Jun 22;12(6):e0178621. doi: 10.1371/journal.pone.0178621. PMID: 28640822; PMCID: PMC5480856.

Chapter 1

Bayer ML, Magnusson SP, Kjaer M; Tendon Research Group Bispebjerg. Early versus delayed rehabilitation after acute muscle injury. *N Engl J Med.* 2017 Sep 28;377(13):1300–1301. doi: 10.1056/NEJMc1708134. PMID: 28953439.

Bennell KL, Ahamed Y, Jull G, et al. Physical therapist-delivered pain coping skills training and exercise for knee osteoarthritis: Randomized controlled trial. *Arthritis Care Res* (Hoboken). 2016 May;68(5):590–602. doi: 10.1002/acr.22744. PMID: 26417720.

Honeyman PT, Jacobs EA. Effects of culture on back pain in Australian aboriginals. *Spine* (Philadelphia 1976). 1996 Apr 1;21(7):841–843. doi: 10.1097/00007632-199604010-00013. PMID: 8779015.

Lin IB, O'Sullivan PB, Coffin JA, Mak DB, Toussaint S, Straker LM. Disabling chronic low back pain as an iatrogenic disorder: A qualitative study in Aboriginal Australians. *BMJ Open.* 2013 Apr 9;3(4):e002654. doi: 10.1136/bmjopen-2013-002654. PMID: 23575999; PMCID: PMC3641505.

Oftedal G, Straume A, Johnsson A, Stovner LJ. Mobile phone headache: A double blind, sham-controlled provocation study. *Cephalalgia.* 2007 May;27(5):447–455. doi: 10.1111/j.1468-2982.2007.01336.x. Epub 2007 Mar 14. PMID: 17359515.

Pollard A, Cronin G. Compression bandaging for soft tissue injury of the ankle: A literature review. *Emerg Nurse.* 2005 Oct;13(6):20–25. doi: 10.7748/en2005.10.13.6.20.c1218. PMID: 16259237.

Chapter 3

Horga LM, Hirschmann AC, Henckel J, et al. Prevalence of abnormal findings in 230 knees of asymptomatic adults using 3.0 T MRI. *Skeletal Radiol.* 2020 Jul;49(7):1099–1107. doi: 10.1007/s00256-020-03394-z. Epub 2020 Feb 14. PMID: 32060622; PMCID: PMC7237395.

Sherman J. *Stone Crusade: A Historical Guide to Bouldering in America.* Golden, CO: American Alpine Club; 1994.

Chapter 4

Inman VT, Saunders JB, Abbott LC. Observations of the function of the shoulder joint. 1944. *Clin Orthop Relat Res.* 1996 Sep;(330):3–12. doi: 10.1097/00003086-199609000-00002. PMID: 8804269.

Jauhiainen S, Pohl AJ, Äyrämö S, Kauppi JP, Ferber R. A hierarchical cluster analysis to determine whether injured runners exhibit similar kinematic gait patterns. *Scand J Med Sci Sports.* 2020 Apr;30(4):732–740. doi: 10.1111/sms.13624. Epub 2020 Jan 22. PMID: 31900980.

Lehman G. Your cranky nerves: A primer for understanding pain. June 10, 2013. https://www.greglehman.ca/blog/2013/06/10/your-cranky -nerves-a-primer-for-patients-to-understand-pain.

May S, Chance-Larsen K, Littlewood C, Lomas D, Saad M. Reliability of physical examination tests used in the assessment of patients with shoulder problems: A systematic review. *Physiotherapy.* 2010 Sep; 96(3):179–190. doi: 10.1016/j.physio.2009.12.002. Epub 2010 Mar 29. PMID: 20674649.

Popper KR. *Realism and the Aim of Science*. London: Hutchinson; 1988.

Talbott JH, Michelsen J. Heat cramps: A clinical and chemical study. *J Clin Invest*. 1933 May;12(3):533–549. doi: 10.1172/JCI100516. PMID: 16694141; PMCID: PMC435921.

Chapter 5

Zulman DM, Haverfield MC, Shaw JG, et al. Practices to foster physician presence and connection with patients in the clinical encounter. *JAMA*. 2020 Jan 7;323(1):70–81. doi: 10.1001/jama.2019.19003. Erratum in: JAMA. 2020 Mar 17;323(11):1098. PMID: 31910284.

Chapter 6

Assa T, Geva N, Zarkh Y, Defrin R. The type of sport matters: Pain perception of endurance athletes versus strength athletes. *Eur J Pain*. 2019 Apr;23(4):686–696. doi: 10.1002/ejp.1335. Epub 2018 Nov 18. PMID: 30379385.

Brady B, Veljanova I, Schabrun S, Chipchase L. Integrating culturally informed approaches into physiotherapy assessment and treatment of chronic pain: A pilot randomised controlled trial. *BMJ Open*. 2018 Jul 5;8(7):e021999. doi: 10.1136/bmjopen-2018-021999. PMID: 29980547; PMCID: PMC6042550.

Dimsdale JE, Dantzer R. A biological substrate for somatoform disorders: Importance of pathophysiology. *Psychosom Med*. 2007 Dec;69(9):850–854. doi: 10.1097/PSY.0b013e31815b00e7. PMID: 18040093; PMCID: PMC2908292.

Elfering A, Mannion AF, Jacobshagen N, Tamcan O, Müller U. Beliefs about back pain predict the recovery rate over 52 consecutive weeks. *Scand J Work Environ Health*. 2009 Dec;35(6):437–445. doi: 10.5271/sjweh.1360. Epub 2009 Oct 2. PMID: 19806279.

Engel GL. The need for a new medical model: A challenge for biomedicine. *Psychodyn Psychiatry*. 2012 Sep;40(3):377–396. doi: 10.1521/pdps.2012.40.3.377. PMID: 23002701.

Wiech K, Farias M, Kahane G, Shackel N, Tiede W, Tracey I. An fMRI study measuring analgesia enhanced by religion as a belief system. *Pain*. 2008 Oct 15;139(2):467–476. doi: 10.1016/j.pain.2008.07.030. Epub 2008 Sep 5. PMID: 18774224.

Chapter 7

Janal MN, Colt EWD, Clark CW, Glusman M. Pain sensitivity, mood and plasma endocrine levels in man following long-distance running: Effects of naloxone. *Pain*. 1984 May;19(1):13–25. doi: 10.1016/0304-3959(84)90061-7. PMID: 6330643.

Chapter 8

Dolce JJ, Crocker MF, Moletteire C, Doleys DM. Exercise quotas, anticipatory concern and self-efficacy expectancies in chronic pain: A preliminary report. *Pain*. 1986 Mar;24(3):365–372. doi: 10.1016/0304-3959(86)90122-3. PMID: 3960576.

Friedman DJ, Khan KM. Preventing overdiagnosis and the harms of too much sport and exercise medicine. *Br J Sports Med*. 2019 Oct;53(20):1314–1318. doi: 10.1136/bjsports-2018-100039. Epub 2018 Dec 5. PMID: 30518520; PMCID: PMC6837247.

Kim H, Lee S. Effects of pain neuroscience education on kinesiophobia in patients with chronic pain: A systematic review and meta-analysis. *Phys Ther Rehabil Sci*. 2020;9:309–317. doi: 10.14474/ptrs.2020.9.4.309.

Larson E. Tackling opioids: Rethinking a "medicalized" approach to pain. LinkedIn. January 31, 2019. https://www.linkedin.com/pulse/tackling-opioids-rethinking-medicalized-approach-pain-eric-b-larson/.

Nicholas MK. The pain self-efficacy questionnaire: Taking pain into account. *Eur J Pain*. 2007 Feb;11(2):153–163. doi: 10.1016/j.ejpain.2005.12.008. Epub 2006 Jan 30. PMID: 16446108.

Parsons T. Illness and the role of the physician: A sociological perspective. *Am J Orthopsychiatry*. 1951;21(3):452–460. doi: 10.1111/j.1939-0025.1951.tb00003.x.

Paterno MV, Flynn K, Thomas S, Schmitt LC. Self-reported fear predicts functional performance and second ACL injury after ACL reconstruction and return to sport: A pilot study. *Sports Health*. 2018 May/Jun;10(3):228–233. doi: 10.1177/1941738117745806. Epub 2017 Dec 22. PMID: 29272209; PMCID: PMC5958451.

Chapter 10

Choi S, Nah S, Jang HD, et al. Association between chronic low back pain and degree of stress: A nationwide cross-sectional study. *Sci Rep*. 2021;11:14549. doi: 10.1038/s41598-021-94001-1.

Dunn WR, Kuhn JE, Sanders R, et al. 2013 Neer Award: Predictors of failure of nonoperative treatment of chronic, symptomatic, full-thickness rotator cuff tears. *J Shoulder Elbow Surg*. 2016 Aug;25(8):1303–1311. doi: 10.1016/j.jse.2016.04.030. PMID: 27422460.

Ingraham P. MRI and X-ray often worse than useless for back pain. Painscience.com. August 27, 2021. https://www.painscience.com/articles/mri-and-x-ray-almost-useless-for-back-pain.php?fbclid=IwAR0HfWXzszmKVikxsj1lgkCq--oaoKqosKclByhfMuygbE2_XeUMPD_zr_E.

Lea M, Hofmann BM. Dediagnosing—a novel framework for making people less ill. *Eur J Intern Med*. 2021 Aug 17:S0953-6205(21)00261-2. doi: 10.1016/j.ejim.2021.07.011. Epub ahead of print. PMID: 34417089.

Lieberthal K, Paterson KL, Cook J, Kiss Z, Girdwood M, Bradshaw EJ. Prevalence and factors associated with asymptomatic Achilles tendon pathology in male distance runners. *Phys Ther Sport*. 2019 Sep; 39:64–68. doi: 10.1016/j.ptsp.2019.06.006. Epub 2019 Jun 17. PMID: 31261019.

O'Sullivan P. It's time for change with the management of non-specific chronic low back pain. *Br J Sports Med*. 2012 Mar;46(4):224–227. doi: 10.1136/bjsm.2010.081638. Epub 2011 Aug 4. PMID: 21821612.

Rajasekaran S, Dilip Chand Raja S, Pushpa BT, Ananda KB, Ajoy Prasad S, Rishi MK. The catastrophization effects of an MRI report on the patient and surgeon and the benefits of "clinical reporting": Results from an RCT and blinded trials. *Eur Spine J.* 2021 Jul;30(7):2069–2081. doi: 10.1007/s00586-021-06809-0. Epub 2021 Mar 21. PMID: 33748882.

Schellingerhout JM, Verhagen AP, Thomas S, Koes BW. Lack of uniformity in diagnostic labeling of shoulder pain: Time for a different approach. *Man Ther.* 2008 Dec;13(6):478–483. doi: 10.1016/j.math.2008.04.005. Epub 2008 Jun 13. PMID: 18555732.

About the Authors

Ryan Whited is a personal trainer, an elite climber, and the founder of Paragon Athletics, a gym that empowers athletes with sport-specific strength and conditioning to complement their performance goals. His passion for working with athletes and investigating the nature of biomechanics and human performance is the basis for Paragon's innovative Training as Treatment program.

Paragon has become a destination for both novice and elite athletes who find themselves sidelined by chronic pain or injury. As a specialist in pain science and physiology, Ryan uses his experience and expertise to help his clients avoid surgery, reduce or eliminate pain, and return to their sports better equipped for the demands required of them.

Ryan lives and trains in Flagstaff, Arizona, with his wife, Betsy, and son, Lane.

Matt Fitzgerald is an acclaimed endurance sports author, coach, and nutritionist. His many books include *The Comeback Quotient*, *80/20 Running*, and *On Pace*. Matt has also written for several leading sports and fitness publications, including *Runner's World* and *Triathlete*, and for popular websites such as outsideonline.com and nbcnews.com.

Matt is a cofounder of 80/20 Endurance, the world's premier endurance sports training brand, and the creator of Dream Run Camp, a pro-style residential training camp for runners of all abilities based in Flagstaff. He also codirects the Coaches of Color Initiative, a nonprofit program that seeks to improve diversity in endurance coaching.

A lifelong endurance athlete, Matt speaks frequently at events throughout the United States and internationally.